"*Fighting for My Life* is a great read. Jamie Tyrone is a champion and a warrior for the millions of people now living with Alzheimer's and future generations who will face this devastating disease. By telling her story honestly, and by courageously volunteering for a clinical trial, Jamie shows the incredible power of one person in the fight for a treatment or cure, and better brain health for all."

—GEORGE VRADENBURG, CHAIRMAN AND
COFOUNDER OF USAGAINSTALZHEIMER'S

"In *Fighting for My Life*, Jamie Tyrone gives a grounded, hopeful, and often humorous account of her diagnosis and commitment to fight back against Alzheimer's. The only way to discover treatments and cures for this insidious and pernicious disease is for heroes like Jamie to volunteer for therapeutic clinical trials. Jamie is performing an incalculable service by sharing her experience as a clinical trial participant. Combining Jamie's personal journey with Dr. Marwan Sabbagh's command of the science and the critical importance of volunteering for Alzheimer's-related trials gives the reader an inspiring and much-needed understanding of one the greatest challenges facing our society today: what it will take to find a cure for Alzheimer's."

—JOHN DWYER, PRESIDENT OF THE GLOBAL
ALZHEIMER'S PLATFORM FOUNDATION

"Rare is the opportunity to delve into the topic of Alzheimer's disease from two different perspectives at the same time. For Jamie Tyrone, the unexpected trauma of finding out she is genetically predisposed to Alzheimer's, and for Dr. Marwan Sabbagh, the insight he's gained from years of research and seeing patients. You may expect their stories to lead to the doom and gloom tale one is often given with anything related to Alzheimer's, but in this case, we are inspired. Tyrone transforms her life to become an advocate, and Sabbagh enlightens us on why there is hope from the medical perspective. If you are one of the millions impacted by Alzheimer's Disease, don't miss the opportunity to read *Fighting For My Life*."

—DEBORAH KAN, FOUNDER AND EXECUTIVE EDITOR OF *BEING
PATIENT*, AWARD-WINNING NEWS ANCHOR AND JOURNALIST, AND
FORMER EXECUTIVE PRODUCER AT THE *WALL STREET JOURNAL*

Praise for *Fighting for My Life*

"For the millions of Americans with Alzheimer's Disease and the millions more who care for them, there has been little hope and much suffering. Until now. *Fighting for My Life* is a remarkable story of hope and possibility for preventing and overcoming this dreaded disease. Dr. Marwan Sabbagh, who leads Cleveland Clinic's efforts to beat this disease, maps out science-based strategies to prevent this disease and improve brain function (for those at risk and the rest of us). If you are a caretaker or at risk for dementia, or if you are anyone with a brain, you must read this book."

—MARK HYMAN, MD, DIRECTOR OF THE CLEVELAND CLINIC
CENTER FOR FUNCTIONAL MEDICINE AND *NEW YORK TIMES*
BESTSELLING AUTHOR OF *FOOD: WHAT THE HECK SHOULD I EAT?*

"To test or not to test is the issue. *Fighting for My Life* is a testament to what happens when someone owns their Alzheimer's risk profile and then teams up with top researchers like Marwan Sabbagh, MD, by signing up for clinical trials. Science needs millions more just like Jamie Tyrone in order to get to a cure."

—MERYL COMER, AUTHOR OF THE *NEW YORK TIMES* BESTSELLER
*SLOW DANCING WITH A STRANGER: LOST AND FOUND IN THE AGE OF
ALZHEIMER'S* AND COFOUNDER OF WOMEN AGAINST ALZHEIMER'S.

"Jamie Tyrone and Dr. Marwan Sabbagh have written an informative and inspiring book to empower those who are exploring their options for genetic testing, deploying strategies for better brain health, and sharing the exciting future of finding a prevention or cure. The only way to eradicate the devastating effects of Alzheimer's Disease is through research and participation in clinical trials. Jamie's courage to share her raw and candid journey of knowing her 91 percent lifetime genetic risk of getting AD, choosing to demystify her selfless experience as a research volunteer, and encouraging others to follow in her footsteps is brave and commendable. *Fighting for My Life* is a compelling must-read."

—JAMES KEACH, AWARD-WINNING DOCUMENTARY PRODUCER
OF *GLEN CAMPBELL: I'LL BE ME* AND *TURNING POINT*

"Jamie Tyrone and Dr. Sabbagh's *Fighting for My Life* punctuates the strength of advocacy to meet the needs of researchers in the quest for finding prevention or a cure through pharmaceutical intervention, early diagnosis, and brain-health strategies. Advocacy does not happen in a vacuum, and this book highlights the true power that using one's voice can have on bringing about positive change in our society. As a supporter in the fight against Alzheimer's Disease, I admire Jamie's dedication to advocacy and Dr. Sabbagh's passion to find a cure."

—Representative John Garamendi

"Participants in clinical research are our heroes. As researchers, our efforts to get new medicines to people around the world could never be achieved without those like Jamie who are willing to join us on the journey. Especially in the case of Alzheimer's Disease, we frequently hear that participating in a clinical trial is empowering and brings hope. We are so thankful to Jamie and Dr. Sabbagh for joining forces to tell this very important story about courage, initiative, and a fighting spirit."

—Phyllis Barkman Ferrell, pharmaceutical executive

"There isn't enough runway for me to express my gratitude to Jamie Tyrone and Dr. Sabbagh for writing this book, or to convey its importance to the fabric of discussions regarding the responsible delivery of genomic medicine. This book should be a guidepost to those who are either considering or ordering predictive genetic testing for Alzheimer's Disease. Jamie is one of many I have heard from who felt emotionally blindsided by their genetic test results because they didn't have the anticipatory guidance to consider how results would make them feel, or the psychiatric and practical struggles they may face. This book has earned its rightful place as one of many to enhance our understanding and guide our individual and collective choices."

—Susan Estabrooks Hahn, MS, LCGC, past president of
the American Board of Genetic Counseling and coauthor
of *Genetic Counseling and Testing for Alzheimer disease:
Joint Practice Guidelines of the American College of Medical
Genetics and the National Society of Genetic Counselors*

Fighting
for My
Life

HOW TO THRIVE IN THE
SHADOW OF ALZHEIMER'S

Jamie TenNapel Tyrone and

Marwan Noel Sabbagh, MD

with John Hanc

W PUBLISHING GROUP

AN IMPRINT OF THOMAS NELSON

Note: some names have been changed throughout this manuscript.

Published in Nashville, Tennessee, by W Publishing, an imprint of Thomas Nelson.

Thomas Nelson titles may be purchased in bulk for educational, business, fund-raising, or promotional use. For information, please e-mail SpecialMarkets@ThomasNelson.com.

Any Internet addresses, phone numbers, or company or product information printed in this book are offered as a resource and are not intended in any way to be or to imply an endorsement by Thomas Nelson, nor does Thomas Nelson vouch for the existence, content, or services of these sites, phone numbers, companies, or products beyond the life of this book.

ISBN 978-0-7852-2155-5 (HC)
ISBN 978-0-7852-2210-1 (SC)
ISBN 978-0-7852-2215-6 (eBook)

Library of Congress Control Number: 2018911311

Printed and bound in the UK using 100% Renewable Electricity at CPI Group (UK) Ltd

To my mother, Suzanne. I continue the fight in your memory and with your unconditional love, strength, and humor to sustain me.
—*Jamie Tyrone*

I dedicate this book to the families and caregivers of my patients. They taught me what love, patience, perseverance, and compassion look like in the face of enduring stress and adversity.
—*Dr. Marwan Sabbagh*

Contents

CONTENTS

Foreword

Have you ever wondered about your genetic risk for Alzheimer's disease?

Or would you rather not know?

Either way, I hope you won't be blindsided by the news, as Jamie Tyrone was when she took a genetic test in an effort to learn her predisposition for a totally unrelated condition. Her accidental discovery of a high risk for Alzheimer's was traumatic, but it propelled Jamie to a journey of self-discovery—a journey that has resulted in this book.

And make no mistake: this book should change your life. If it doesn't, you either didn't need to read it because you are diligently making all the right choices and enjoying them, or because you just don't understand how much control you have over your brain's long-term health.

Thankfully, Dr. Sabbagh and Jamie know that oftentimes knowledge isn't enough. As you read, you'll laugh, cry, and experience the anger and other raw emotions Jamie experienced once she truly understood the risks involved for her future. You can't help but connect with Jamie as you read her story—and you'll rejoice when you see how that story led her to Marwan Sabbagh, MD, the person I consider to be the "go to" doc when it comes to treating and researching Alzheimer's disease and other forms of dementia.

While Alzheimer's and all the dementias can be devastating to individuals and their families, the good news is that you can take actions now that will radically delay or maybe even stop you from developing the condition. The double-4 genotype that was so devastating to Jamie years ago may not have to be so devastating in today's world.

That's the incredible message of this book: you have power. You can change your future.

As Dr. Sabbagh and Jamie Tyrone make clear, you have a great chance to change which of your genes are "turned on" and which are not. Incredibly, you have the ability to change your family history going forward. In addition to Jamie's story, this book will help you by detailing the science behind how to make those choices that will radically diminish your future risk for dementia.

That's where Dr. Sabbagh's influence is critical within these pages. Independent of and irrespective to your specific genes, he describes at least ten choices you can make that will delay or diminish the onset of dementia. These ten choices are important for all of us, given that dementia risk increases the longer we live. And all of us are living longer. In fact, you are likely (very likely as we move into the 2020s) to live past eighty-five—the age when a third of us develop dementia. Thankfully, while medical science is enabling us to live longer, it also, with the help of great scientists such as Dr. Sabbagh, is enabling us to make choices that make dementia much less likely.

As you'll see in these pages, those choices can be as simple as routine stress management; doing specific physical activities and specific brain games; having lots of friends you rely on and associating with them frequently; avoiding toxins such as mercury and tobacco; avoiding unforced errors such as not wearing a helmet when skiing; making diet choices such as ensuring adequate brain fats, coffee, nuts, and chocolate; and the easiest choice of all, taking some especially helpful supplements.

Dr. Sabbagh sheds light on these choices and many others you can make *right now* to delay or diminish dementia.

Having these choices is a wonderful gift. But be aware there is a paradox connected to them—having a choice doesn't always lead to better decisions.

For example, you would think that having an increased risk of a disease such as Alzheimer's would lead a person to make better choices for preventing that disease. But that's not always the case. As you'll see in Jamie's emotional and engaging story, things get complicated. Fear must be overcome.

I'm grateful for the choices Jamie has made in recent years to fight back against the shadow of Alzheimer's—to fight not only for her own future, but for yours as well. I'm also grateful for the contributions of Dr. Sabbagh both to this book and to our general knowledge of the science between the important choices described in these pages.

So please take advantage of these pages. If you want to understand the science behind Alzheimer's and other forms of dementia, this book is for you. If you want to understand the choices you can make to delay or work toward preventing the onset of such dementia, this book is for you. And if you are interested in a powerful and emotional story of hope, this book is certainly for you.

Before I close, I want to make a special mention of the sections in this book written specifically for caregivers. I have seen the way dementia ravages not just individuals, but whole families. I've watched the difficulty of those struggling with caregiving. This book makes that easier, which is an incredible contribution.

I'm not surprised by that contribution, of course. The Cleveland Clinic's Lou Ruvo Center for Brain Health—led by Dr. Sabbagh—was founded by friends of a man who watched his torment as he cared lovingly and consistently for his father. Though the process took a toll on him, he recovered with the help of science, his choices, and his family and friends. Jamie and Marwan point out that up to 40 percent of caregivers die prior to the ones they are caring for. Thus, caregivers need to make great choices and care for themselves too.

As you'll see, Jamie and Marwan not only reveal the secrets of caregiving for a person entering and living with dementia (the caregiver and the patient both live with dementia), but also how to minimize the risks to the caregiver and improve the care of the loved one in the process. Let me repeat—this section is outstanding. It's the best material on caregiving I've seen in any book on Alzheimer's or the dementias, and it's especially important if the caregiver is expected to help both himself and the one cared for escape the ravages of dementia.

And you can escape. That's the power and knowledge this book puts in your hands.

Finally, don't just read this book. Take action. Make the choices Jamie and Marwan have shared in these pages. Those choices will make you a better caregiver, yes. But those choices may keep *your* loved ones from ever having to be a caregiver. That's exactly what's at stake.

—Dr. Michael Roizen

Introduction

Where was she?

Where was Grandma Neva?

I scanned the room, searching through my ten-year-old eyes for this woman I'd never met but pictured clearly in my mind. Based on what I'd heard about her, how she had been born on a farm in the late 1800s and taught in a one-room schoolhouse, I imagined Grandma Neva looking like a cross between *Whistler's Mother* and Auntie Em from *The Wizard of Oz*—with a little Annie Oakley thrown in.

Such a person was nowhere to be found amidst the adults who had crowded into the parlor of my aunt Opal's house to welcome travelers from a distant coast. My disappointment at not seeing the mythical grandmother was quickly overcome by the sheer excitement of being their center of attention. "Aren't you a pretty little thing?" my aunt Opal said as she smothered me with a hug.

To a ten-year-old girl from the suburbs of Los Angeles, this strange new land called Iowa was filled with curious and magical sights.

What were those giant stalks I saw through Aunt Opal's window, shooting skyward in the distance? Corn, really? Like the stuff in the Green Giant can? Why were the men wearing overalls? And how did they get so tan with no beaches around?

There were warm and delicious smells, as well; chickens roasting, kernels frying, apple pies—made especially by my aunt Opal for our arrival—baking hot and crisp and sweet.

The arrival of my mom, her husband, and three children was big news in Keokuk County. This was where my mom, Suzanne, had spent part of her childhood. Still, amidst the parade of relatives I was meeting for the first time—uncles, aunts, second and third cousins I never knew existed—what was puzzling was the absence of the family matriarch, the saintly old woman whose face I searched for in vain: Neva Williams Finch, my great-grandmother.

Pronounced "Nee-va," the name alone sounded exotic and alluring. Popular for girls in the late nineteenth century—she was born in 1883—Neva is supposedly Latin for "snow," of which I was told they got plenty of in Keokuk County. But not now. It was the summer of 1971, and we had driven there from far-off LA. And it was during that trip that I learned the story of Grandma Neva.

My memories of her were really my mother's: Neva was *her* grandmother, and they had spent considerable time together when, sometimes for months, she had been conveniently deposited in the Midwest by her mother, Ethel—an Iowa native who had moved to California as a young woman. While Ethel and her first husband "worked things out" (presumably a 1940s way of saying that they were getting a divorce), my mom was inaugurated into the traditional, uncluttered rhythms of agrarian life with Grandma Neva.

Now Suzanne was returning for the first time in years. My dad, a professional truck driver, sat behind the wheel of the family station wagon during the three-day trip, the muted sounds of American Top 40 radio—Carole King's "It's Too Late," the pre-disco Bee Gees' "How Can You Mend a Broken Heart?" and James Taylor's "You've Got a Friend"— droning in and out through a hiss of static and a series of changing stations as we plunged into the heartland. We clocked 1,763 miles from

California through Utah, Colorado, Nebraska, and to the southeast corner of Iowa, where rural Keokuk County is located.

In the back seat, my eight-year-old brother, Don, and thirteen-year-old sister, Lisa, and I fought and bickered. Partly to quiet us down, but mostly I think because she wanted to relive and share her precious memories, my mom told us stories of her time with Grandma Neva, unrolling her recollections as the miles clicked off on the Ford's odometer.

"Grandma Neva was a teacher," she told us.

Where?

"In a one-room schoolhouse."

What? No way!

"It's true. And she was also a farmer's wife."

Did he have a scarecrow?

"Probably. They grew corn and beans, and that's what they ate for dinner."

Yuck. No hamburgers?

"Oh, the food on the farm was delicious. You'll see."

What did you do with Grandma Neva when you were little?

"We'd sit on the porch and shuck corn and peas."

Shuck?

"That means you'd peel them." Mom would then manipulate her hands in the air, demonstrating a skill that was as foreign to us in 1971 as dialing a rotary phone would be to kids today.

"She also taught me to play the zither."

The what-er?

Again, using her hands, Mom demonstrated the quaint stringed instrument, popular among American families when Neva was growing up. I could almost hear the mournful sounds of those plucked, brittle notes.

As Mom told her rich stories of life with Neva, I thought of an old book I'd found in the children's section of our public library in Glendale, part of a series that would soon become a popular TV show.

Was this like Little House on the Prairie?

"Kind of. You couldn't just turn on a faucet to get water. You had to walk out to a well. And there was no electricity—and no bathroom."

This news was particularly alarming to my thirteen-year-old sister. *What do you mean "no bathroom"?*

"You had to use an outhouse."

What's that?

"Well, basically, it's a bathroom out in the backyard."

Gross!

Recalling that 1971 trip, my mom still chuckles when she thinks of those conversations with her kids about her own childhood. "And Jamie," she'll say to me, "you were so disappointed when we got to Aunt Opal's and found out that now they had running water and regular bathrooms."

It was the day after we'd arrived when I finally heard Grandma Neva's name mentioned by someone other than my mother. I remember the effect it had. What had been a convivial conversation around Aunt Opal's dining room table suddenly grew somber. Sitting nearby, I strained to discern what the adults presumably didn't want us kids to hear. I picked up an unfamiliar phrase. Something about arteries that were hardening. I had no idea what that meant. Then, my uncle Buck, a loveable rogue, put down his glass and stood up. "She's gotten old, Suzanne," he said to my mom with a shrug. "Fact of life. Happens to all of us, right?" He spotted me nearby. "Hey tadpole," he said, brightening. "You wanna go try and catch some more walleye?"

I did, and off we went in his truck, probably—well almost certainly—not buckling our seat belts. If he even had them.

The next morning, Mom announced that we were going to visit Grandma Neva. "We are?" I exclaimed. "That's great!"

Mom smiled thinly and nodded. She didn't seem to think it was so great, which struck me as odd. Didn't she want to see this person she'd been telling us about for days?

That afternoon, we piled into the car and drove to the outskirts of town. My brother and sister, some of our cousins, my mom, and Aunt Opal. We kids were buzzing and chirping in the back until Opal steered the car into the parking lot of what looked like a hospital.

"We're going to see Grandma Neva in her home" is what we had been told on the way.

This sure doesn't look very homey, I thought.

We walked in and were immediately assaulted by the stench of urine, an odor pervasive and strong enough to make me gag. The smell affected me so much that a decade or so later, when I was a nursing student choosing a specialty, I opted for the OR, where you see plenty of blood but are generally spared the scent of urine.

Despite the overpowering smell, I straightened up and was mindful of not making a scene. We were meeting Grandma Neva, after all, and I wanted to make a good impression on the woman who meant so much to my mom and whom I felt like I knew, thanks to Mom's enchanting stories.

I'd rehearsed in my mind my greeting and the many questions I had for her: "Hello, Grandma Neva, I'm Jamie TenNapel, your great-granddaughter. I live in California. Can you still play the zither? Do you think you might come visit us sometime? I'd like you to see me play tennis."

If time permitted, I'd go on and ask her to tell me some stories about growing up. Did she ever see any cowboys or Indians for real? Did they have animals on the farm? What were their names? Oh, and what about that outhouse?

As we walked down the corridor, I saw people sitting in wheelchairs, arrayed along the wall. Now I should say here that in all likelihood, by the conventions of what were then called "rest" or "old age" homes, this one was probably up to code and, for the standards of the time, compassionately run. Yet it seemed to me as grim and gothic as a Dickensian workhouse. Part of it was simply the fact that for the first time I was coming face-to-face with old age at its worst, with senility, and, although few knew it then, with Alzheimer's disease.

Trying to be friendly, I wanted to say hello to an old gentleman as we walked through the lobby, but he seemed to be looking right through me. His jaw was slack; his expression startled, as if being placed in this corridor and his wheelchair was all a big surprise to him. He also had on him what looked like a harness—a Posey vest which, I would learn in nursing school, is used to restrain patients who might fall out of their wheelchair.

I turned to my mom. "Is this, like, a jail?"

"No!" she said firmly and then paused, seeming to search for the right answer. "It's . . . well, it's a home for old folks."

That word again. *Home.* Did people have to be tied to chairs in their own home? And why did all the people I passed look the way they did—glassy-eyed, uncommunicative, and for the most part silent? As we walked past the reception desk and down the corridor, my aunt leading the way, I did hear laughter and talking. *Finally, some signs of life!* I thought. I sneaked a peek and saw a woman in her wheelchair, facing a wall—conversing with no one.

We came to a nurses station, the kids having gathered closer to the adults. Even my cool sister seemed a bit spooked.

Opal and my mom asked the nurses about Neva's whereabouts, not that anyone was worried she might have decided to fly to New York for the weekend on a whim. Sadly, as I was beginning to understand, the boundaries of her life, like all of those here, had been reduced to those gray institutional walls.

"Neva?" asked one of the nurses. "Oh, we have her in the day room."

That sounded promising: someplace lighter and more airy than the dark hallways we'd just walked through. Someplace where perhaps they could open the windows and let in some fresh air.

But when we walked in, it was more of the same. More elderly people, a few sitting erect, most of them slouched over as if gravity was pulling them to the grave that, for many, might have been a blessing. I looked around. In the corner, a stack of worn board games—Monopoly, Parcheesi, a checkers set—unused. A black-and-white TV with the sound down. Much to my chagrin, the smell was just as potent. But it was here that I finally saw Grandma Neva—from the back at first—a whirl of white hair sprouting out of a wheelchair. My aunt and mom went around to face her and then beckoned us to follow.

"Hello, Grandma," I heard my mother saying as she took the withered hand in hers. "Do you remember me?"

When I walked over and turned to face her, my knees trembled. This wasn't the strong, skilled, and intelligent woman I'd envisioned. This wasn't someone who could teach you how to shuck corn or play a musical instrument, much less read or write.

Grandma Neva was slouched in her chair, a line of drool snaking down her chin and on to a soiled hospital gown. Her eyes were dim behind smudged spectacles, her mouth agape. She, too, wore a restraint. She, too, reeked of urine.

I don't recall being introduced. It wouldn't have mattered. It was clear even to a ten-year-old that there would be no conversations, no questions, no discussion of trips and visits.

Years later, my mom would tell me that Neva had actually responded to her that day. "You're Glenn Stover's girl," she'd rasped, correctly identifying the name of my mother's father.

Somehow, hearing that made it almost worse for me. It meant that Neva might have had some flicker of consciousness, some dim awareness of her surroundings—of the sodden, humiliating, inescapable situation she was in. That to me was all the more horrifying. As was the fact that she would live in that wretched condition—if you could call it living—for six more years.

Neva White eventually died in that same nursing home in January 1977. She was ninety-three.

<hr />

The car was silent as we drove back to Aunt Opal's that day. And although I would go on to have a wonderful time during the rest of our two-week-long Midwest trip, I wrestled for some time afterward with occasional nightmares about Grandma Neva and the nursing home, until the specters of leering, wrinkled faces and wheelchairs chasing me down corridors eventually receded deep in my cerebral cortex.

Thirty-eight years later it all came roaring back.

This time, it was I who sat slack-jawed. It was April 2009, and I was staring at my computer screen in my home office in Ramona, California.

What I had just googled had left me bloodless and numb. A few months earlier, I had agreed to participate in a genetic study, similar to the popular 23andMe tests. This particular study was designed to assess how subjects would react if they knew they were at an increased risk of getting a disease. Would they change their lifestyle, knowing they were harboring a genetic time bomb?

Turns out I was harboring such a bomb. And it appeared to have just blown up in my face.

Based on the results I had been e-mailed, followed by a quick check on a website to try and interpret the woefully inadequate information I had received along with those results, I learned that I had inherited two genes I had never heard of—called ApoE4—one from each parent.

This put me at a 91 percent lifetime risk of contracting Alzheimer's disease—almost a guarantee. And for those with this particular genetic signature, the average age for onset of the disease is sixty-five.

Imagine reading that about yourself. How would you feel? What would you do?

The story of how I reacted—of how this news affected me; the depths to which I descended as the notion of such a grim, preordained fate took hold of me; my desperate and often fruitless search for help; and how I eventually found it through good people like my coauthor, Dr. Marwan Sabbagh, of the Cleveland Clinic—well, that's what this book is about.

In these pages Dr. Sabbagh, one of the country's leading experts on what those who study and treat Alzheimer's disease call "AD," will explain the science behind this devastating and increasingly prevalent disease.

I will tell you how I fought—how I'm still fighting—for my life and for my future.

Dr. Sabbagh and I will both offer some thoughts on how genetic testing like this for AD, so common now, has changed—and needs to change even more. And just as important, at an exciting time in research on AD, we'll tell you about some of the things you can do to fight back—for yourself or a loved one.

Hopefully you don't have a 91 percent chance of getting this dreaded condition, but chances are high that the disease will impact you or someone you love in some fashion. According to the Alzheimer's Association, a new case of the disease develops every sixty-five seconds in the United States, a rate that is expected to double in the decades ahead as our population continues to age. The National Institutes of Health now ranks AD as the sixth leading cause of death in this country. Moreover, AD is the only disease in the top ten that cannot be cured, prevented, or slowed.

We need to add the word *yet* to the end of that sentence though. As

Dr. Sabbagh will explain a little later, we are on the precipice of major breakthroughs in treatment, and most experts agree that, while they can't yet pinpoint the mechanism or establish causality, there are things you can do that can likely minimize, delay, and perhaps even prevent this most feared of diseases.

Fear. That's a big part of AD. Fear of getting it, fear of the state it will leave you in, fear of having to care for someone with it. All well-founded fears, as I can attest to. I was paralyzed with dread that night in 2009 as I read the chilling statistic that seemed to foretell my genetic destiny. And amidst the flood of emotions coursing through my brain was a dark, almost primal childhood fear that resurfaced after many dormant decades. As a forty-nine-year-old that night, I was traumatized thinking it would be just a matter of time before I, too, was sitting, restrained and drooling, in a wheelchair.

Now at fifty-eight I'm proud to say I've put my fears aside, and I'm pushing back against my genetic destiny. I'm a full-time advocate for Alzheimer's research and for those who are struggling with family members afflicted by AD. I am the founder of a nonprofit called B.A.B.E.S.—Beating Alzheimer's by Embracing Science—and a founding member of WA2—Women Against Alzheimer's—a movement of women campaigning for new approaches to research the disease that affects females disproportionately and crusading for the adoption of a national plan for the prevention and treatment of AD.

Back in April 2009, a plan was what I urgently needed. My hope is that the stories I share and the information Dr. Sabbagh contributes within this book will help you build your own plan to fight AD, whether for your own life or for those walking alongside others who are fighting for their lives.

CHAPTER 1

A Question of Balance

G ary was dead.

One minute he'd been alive, saying how glad he was to be getting out of the hospital and headed home. The next minute, I turned around and he had stopped breathing and was turning blue.

It was the spring of 1979, and it was my very first day in the hospital. I was in my freshman year as a nursing student at Glendale Community College, and after a semester of class learning I was now starting my clinical rotations at a local hospital. Forget about performing CPR; I could barely make a bed at this point.

Gary was my patient, my very first patient, precisely because he didn't require anything more difficult than to be helped out of bed and given a bath in preparation for his release. Ten days earlier he'd had surgery to remove a benign tumor in his brain. The situation was serious, yes, but he had seemed to make a full recovery. I'd given him his bath and had just helped him into a chair in his hospital room.

We were chatting, and then suddenly we weren't.

I was nineteen at the time. I ran out the door to the nurses station. "Oh my God, oh my God, he's stopped breathing!"

The experienced staff burst into action. Within seconds of calling Code Blue, crash carts were barreling into the room and an internist was attempting to resuscitate him.

I cowered in a corner, praying they could save him.

They couldn't. It was later determined the cause of death was not a poorly administered bath by a clueless student nurse, as I irrationally feared. Gary had died from a pulmonary embolism, which is a blood clot in the lung.

I'd never even seen a dead body before. I stared at Gary's corpse, now turning a slate gray color as it was loaded onto a gurney. One hour earlier, the man was talking to me.

I killed him! the voice in my head said. *This was my fault.*

Just as they were wheeling Gary out, one of my college nursing instructors arrived, who had been alerted as well.

"Jamie," she said, taking me in her arms, "I'm really sorry."

She ushered me into a nearby staff room, put her hands on my shoulder, and looked me in the eye. "You did nothing wrong here," she said. "There was nothing you could have done to have prevented it."

"I . . . I know. But one minute he was alive, and the next minute. . . . And his poor wife."

"Jamie," my instructor said, repeating my name more emphatically. "I think you're going to make a good nurse, but you're going to have to learn that these things happen all the time in hospitals, despite our best efforts. You just have to move on."

I nodded and wiped my eyes with a Kleenex.

"I know it's hard, especially the first time you see it," she continued. "Nobody likes losing a patient. So tell you what, if you'd like to take the day off tomorrow, that's fine with me. Relax. Go to the beach. Hang out with your friends. Just forget about this. And we'll see you back here in two days."

I thanked her. In a daze I left the hospital and drove back to the apartment I shared with two other nursing students. By the time I got home, I'd made up my mind. I was not going to take a day off. It was a kind offer, but it wasn't the way I needed to deal with this. I remember the shopworn but graphic way I used to explain my thinking to one of my roommates: "I just got kicked off the horse. I've got to get back on that horse tomorrow."

I showed up at the hospital the next morning.

TRAUMA CITY

Now fast-forward four years, and I was a registered nurse, working in the operating room of one of LA's busiest trauma centers.

The day Gary died, I'd learned something more than a lesson in the harsh realities of life in a hospital. I'd learned that tenacity was in my makeup, and I could pick myself up after being dealt a body blow. The lesson was an important one and would extend beyond my nursing career. Years later, when *I* became the patient and it was *my* life that was seemingly in jeopardy, the memories of that first day in the hospital and how I dealt with it would help me stay strong. And later still, when I was brought to my knees by the revelation that my illness turned out not to be what I thought it was but something even more terrifying, it was my resilience, my ability to get back on the horse, that eventually saved my life.

After I graduated and passed my nursing boards, I went to work in the OR at California Hospital Medical Center. "Welcome to the Knife and Gun Club," the head nurse said the first day I reported for duty.

That was the nickname the staff had for the hospital. It was my first taste of the dark humor that pervaded the world of the OR—and that probably helped keep everybody sane.

Founded in 1887, California Hospital was already nearly a century old by the time I started there, and it had a reputation of being one of the best trauma centers in the West. Located in an imposing red building on South Grand Avenue, we were in the heart of LA, and this was the early 1980s, the height of the crack epidemic. Victims of gunshot wounds and stabbings were a nightly occurrence for us. I can't tell you how many codes I went through nor the wide range of grievous injuries we saw on a nightly basis, but it was a thrill to be part of a highly skilled, competent team. Everyone knew their job and did it, very often in situations where someone's life depended on it. And we saved far more patients than we lost.

I thought I was pretty tough by that point. Growing up I had been labeled, in the parlance of the day, a "tom girl." I loved sports, especially tennis, which I played throughout high school. But I also participated in sports that girls of that era weren't supposed to play, like football. My mother still has a yellowed clipping from a Glendale newspaper about a flag football game in which I scored a touchdown and was praised for my defensive play as well.

That was me: a two-way threat.

Emotionally, I was sensitive, compassionate, and—since that incident on my first day in the hospital—tenacious. As a nurse in a major inner-city trauma center, I had to learn to dial down the compassion. Given the level of human suffering we saw, not only in the OR where the patients were often grievously injured but also in the hallways and the waiting rooms, I had to learn to keep my emotions in check. Otherwise I would have been unable to function. Any squeamishness or prudishness vanished in the OR as well, as did any sense that people are somehow different.

It seems unusual and even trite in today's diverse world, but growing up in lily white Glendale in the 1970s, I'd not had much contact with people of color. At California Hospital Medical Center, the staff, the docs, the patients, the cops, and the EMTs were all as diverse as the city. My friends and colleagues included African Americans, Mexicans, Central Americans, Koreans, Vietnamese, Chinese, Micronesians, Iranians, Indians, and Pakistanis.

From those we treated, I learned that everyone bled; everyone felt pain, gratitude, and relief. But no matter how bad their circumstances might have seemed, they all wanted to keep on living.

That, of course, was our priority in the OR: keep 'em alive. And we did a good job of it under harrowing circumstances. One of my specialties as a surgical nurse was craniotomies, in which a bone flap is temporarily removed so that the brain can be accessed. Many of these procedures at California Hospital were done as the result of blows to the head or gunshot wounds. But one of the most memorable was a patient who had an aneurism, a bulging blood vessel in the brain. The surgeon removed the bone, with me assisting, but as he began to work on the brain, the patient started hemorrhaging and blood began pooling out all over his brain. He could have perished in minutes. A serious but routine procedure was now an emergency. The surgeon was cool though. He calmly issued instructions as he adroitly clamped the blood vessel. I handed him the surgical patties to absorb the blood in order to clear his field so he could clearly see what he was doing. There was no panic, not even a sense of urgency in his voice. The patient survived. I was proud to be an OR nurse that night and to have been a part of that team.

There were other, less noble moments, but ones that would have a lasting effect on me.

Once, an elderly patient with a broken hip came to the OR for surgery. Part of my job was to do an initial assessment. As the floor nurse handed her off to me in a pre-op holding area, she thought something might be amiss. "I was moving the patient and something sharp hit my hand," she said.

Uh-oh, I thought. That could mean the bone had been displaced and was starting to poke through the skin. If that was the case, it could quickly become infected. I had noticed also in her lab work that the patient had a high potassium level. That could be dangerous to the heart and normally might have meant canceling the operation, but with an open fracture, surgery couldn't be delayed, regardless.

I went to the surgeon and anesthesiologist, who had also seen her lab work. "We're postponing that surgery," the surgeon told me. "Her potassium's high."

I told them my concern and that they might want to reconsider. "I think we're the ones who make that decision," said the anesthesiologist dismissively.

"Doctor," I said, addressing the surgeon, "I think she might have opened her fracture."

Still, both of them seemed reluctant. They didn't want to listen to a young nurse. But this was my responsibility; I was supposed to be the patient's advocate. And in this case, the patient was elderly, semiconscious, and in a potentially dire situation.

"Fine," I said. "Don't operate. But I'm going to the charge nurse, and I'm going to tell her the situation, and then you can deal with her."

They didn't want that hassle. "All right, all right," said the surgeon. "You don't need to make a federal case out of it."

I followed them back to the pre-op area. The physician examined the patient as the anesthesiologist stood by—smirking and presumably waiting to see me embarrassed when I was proven wrong. Then the examining doctor stopped short. I saw him move his hands around her hip.

"Oh," he said. "We need to get her into the OR right now."

The operation was successful and the patient lived. Did anyone—in particular, those two physicians—thank me or the floor nurse who had first noticed the problem? No. But in retrospect that was okay. It was a big deal for me, for any of us excepting the most senior nurses, to challenge a surgeon. For once, I'd used my voice. It was a good lesson. And it wouldn't be the last time I'd have to stand my ground in the face of obstinate, arrogant medical authority.

Still, the stress of working in a big city trauma center night after night wore on people. I could see it on the lined faces of the longtime OR nurses and some of the senior techs. Many of them were cynical, bitter. About the doctors. About the patients. About the health-care system. About life in general. I didn't want to become that way.

The answer could have been my transferring to a hospital in a quiet suburban area; or changing into a new nursing specialty—maybe postpartum, where I'd spend my days in maternity wards filled with happy moms and newborns. But I had a better idea. Every hospital is visited regularly by sales reps from various firms. They're selling everything from needles to X-ray machines to cafeteria food to computer services. While it's often the decision makers in the so-called "c-suite" that they ultimately have to convince, the reps know that it's good to get the staff on their side.

On a regular basis, we'd meet the medical product reps. They'd come into the staff room or drop by the locker rooms. Very often they were former nurses themselves. But they were always stylishly dressed and carried briefcases, like attorneys or physicians. They'd also come armed with boxes of doughnuts or chocolates.

This appealed to my twenty-seven-year-old self. *That's what I want to do*, I thought. *Wear something other than these shapeless scrubs, carrying a briefcase like a professional, and hand out doughnuts to make everyone feel good.* I was already a people pleaser. This seemed perfect!

I didn't realize then that these perky reps were being nice to us because it was part of the sales process. After we were all oohing and aahing and fighting over who got the jelly-filled doughnut or the ones with sprinkles, these sales professionals would give us a brief presentation about their product. Sometimes the sell was even more subtle, done in silky smooth fashion.

"Jamie, you like the honey-glazed ones?" a rep asked me one afternoon, after she'd dropped by our staff room with several boxes of doughnuts.

"Hmpfff," I'd reply, my mouth full as I nodded affirmatively.

"I'm glad," the rep would say, flashing a dazzling white smile. "Hey, you work in the OR, right? So did I. You're starting to use a lot of scopes, aren't you? Did you ever see these?"

She was referring to the new generation of laparoscopic tools that were about to reshape medicine. And she showed me the latest one. It was fine-tuned, light, easier for the physicians to wield than the current models. Of course, I wasn't going to be performing surgery. But we were well trained enough to recognize a superior instrument when we saw it. The rep wanted the nurses to learn about it too. Maybe we'd even drop a word about it to the doctors.

While I might not have appreciated the subtle techniques at first, I knew that being a medical sales rep looked a lot more fun than taking a rectal temperature. In 1987, I left the hospital for a job in a medical sales firm in the LA area. Along with a new job, I decided to get a new look. My blonde, Farrah Fawcett hairdo was out: I dyed my hair fiery red, cut it shorter, and never looked back.

I sold a catalog of products, everything from wound care dressings to catheters. I started by selling to a couple of local hospitals, learned where all the closest doughnut shops were, and did well. Soon I was promoted to district sales manager. It was the beginning of a career that would later land me in the position of marketing director for a large hospital. And eventually, I was the director of business development for the entire Western United States at one of the country's largest long-term, acute-care hospital systems.

But as the saying goes, I had to learn to walk before I could run. And at that point in time, walking had started to become a problem.

LOSING CONTROL

One morning in 1985, shortly before my career switch, as I was walking out the door of my apartment on my way to work, I realized I couldn't control my legs. It was like driving a car where the steering wheel is suddenly and terrifyingly unresponsive.

As I tried to walk straight down the driveway, my legs would veer to the right. I just seemed to be flopping along, as if I were intoxicated or wearing clown shoes. I made it to my car and sat behind the wheel, panting. *What's going on?* I thought. At first, I considered driving myself to the local ER. But by the time I arrived in my office, my legs and gait were back to normal.

Odd, I thought.

Things got scarier one morning a few weeks later when I woke up and couldn't move. I was paralyzed. I could talk; I could have screamed for help, but no one would have come to help me. By now, I had been able to move into my own place. With no roommates to come and rescue me, I lay in bed wondering if this was how I would be found days later and what kind of reaction it might provoke.

I could just picture the headline in the feisty *Los Angeles Examiner*:

GOOD NIGHT, NURSE! RN
FOUND DEAD IN BED!

After about five minutes, I regained all feelings below my neck and simply got out of bed and went about my day as if nothing had happened.

A fluke, I guessed. Maybe it was something in the pasta sauce?

When both symptoms returned a few weeks later, I knew this had nothing to do with anything I was eating or drinking. Also, my right arm was starting to feel weak. I'm a lefty, so I was still able to write, but I could barely pick up my briefcase or my samples.

I had to get this looked at.

"Ataxia," said the neurologist, after he'd listened to my symptoms and examined me. A lack of muscle control or coordination of voluntary movements. There was a long list of possible causes, but the MRI was negative. It could be a symptom of something more serious. Or it could be nothing. "I'm not really sure what's going on," he admitted with a shrug.

Great. Well, I went on with my life, although it was a life in which I had to put up with sudden bouts of instability and loss of control. Once after the end of an important meeting sitting around a conference room table with a client, I got up, felt the strange numb sense of losing control of my legs, and promptly fell right on my bottom.

Appalled, I tried to make a joke out of it. "I didn't have that many glasses of wine last night," I joked. There were a few nervous chuckles in response. "Seriously," I said, as a colleague helped me up. "It happens sometimes. But I've been checked and I'm okay."

Inside, however, I knew I was not okay. One weekend in 1989, while I was sitting out in the sun by a friend's lakeside house, I suddenly felt as if I were detached from the deck chair and floating in air. It was my first case of vertigo. The doctor who examined me suggested that it had probably been triggered by exposure to the sun, which, considering I lived in Southern California, was going to be a hard trigger to avoid.

It went on like that for several years. Weeks, sometimes even months, of nothing. Then, suddenly, a day came when I couldn't control my body—a morning when I couldn't move. An attack of vertigo. What in heaven's name was going on? I decided to find out. In the pre-Internet age it meant some trips to the local library. I also queried my medical colleagues.

Poor balance, difficulty walking, dizziness, heat intolerance, vertigo, muscle rigidity. All classic symptoms of MS: multiple sclerosis.

My friend Susie had been diagnosed with MS a few years earlier. I told her my story and confessed that I was at a dead end. "I'm lost and confused, and I'm not sure where to go next."

"I don't know if you've got MS or not, Jamie," she said. "But I know somebody who will. My doctor; he's the guru of MS."

His name was Dr. Stanley van den Noort, a neurologist at UC-Irvine and chief medical officer at the National Multiple Sclerosis Society.

Many years later in his obituary, the *Los Angeles Times* would hail Dr. van den Noort as a "compassionate" physician and a titan in his specialty; a physician and researcher who, in the words of one of his colleagues, helped build "awareness, understanding and support for speeding us towards a world free of multiple sclerosis."

When I went to visit Dr. van den Noort about my condition, I found him to be all those things: compassionate, authoritative, and a distinguished-looking man who clearly knew his subject.

After examining me, he confirmed that I had many of the classic symptoms, plus one that had just developed: optic neuritis, blurriness in my right eye.

But the results of my MRI were negative. There were no signs of the white brain lesions that are a telltale indicator of MS.

At the conclusion of the examination, Dr. van den Noort and I sat down in his office. "I think you have MS," he said. "However, it could be very early in the process. That would explain why your MRI is normal, but you have most of the other symptoms."

I felt relieved in one sense. Finally, an answer. But then the reality: I had MS. "What do I need to do?"

"You're young, Jamie. You've got a lot of years ahead of you," he said. "Live your life to the fullest."

I knew what he meant. It seemed likely that I had the beginnings of a debilitating disease of the central nervous system, one that could eventually leave me unable to walk. I'd better make hay while the sun was still shining. For the next three years, I tried to follow Dr. van den Noort's advice as my symptoms waxed and waned. I was doing well in hospital marketing. Aside from the occasional fall, I could hide my symptoms pretty well in an office environment, but I was now in my thirties, and like a lot of single, childless women that age I heard both matrimonial and biological clocks ticking.

Who was going to want to marry me now? Who would want a wife who's probably going to be in a wheelchair in a few years? So I developed some guidelines concerning that. If I met a guy I liked, somebody I thought I could possibly get serious with, I'd tell him about my condition on the third date. I knew that would separate the men from the boys. And it usually did.

My luck in that area changed in 1996. By that time, I was thirty-six years old and climbing the ranks of one of the largest long-term, acute-care hospital corporations in the country. I'd rapidly gone from sales to marketing and was now an associate administrator of a facility that we were opening in San Diego. We needed a director of cardiopulmonary services. Of all the candidates for the job, the one I was most impressed with was a former respiratory therapist named Doug Tyrone. He had a solid resume, and when I interviewed him I must admit that I was taken by his really cute smile. More importantly, he seemed like the right man for the job. He was hired.

About five months after he started, I was promoted to the position of corporate regional director. Doug was promoted to take my place. I was happy for him and felt validated in hiring him. But while I saw him around the office and shared occasional small talk about our jobs, there was no longer any reporting relationship. When he asked me out to dinner one night, I said yes.

Doug was twelve years older than I was and had three children from a previous marriage. He was tall, handsome, mustachioed, and had a hilarious sense of humor. I really liked him, and on our third date I knew I had to tell him about my health, and hoped, hoped, hoped his response would be different from the others'.

At a Mexican restaurant in La Jolla, I took a sip of my margarita, followed by a deep breath. "Doug, I think you need to know something about me." He raised an eyebrow. "A couple of years ago, I was diagnosed with MS."

He didn't appear shocked when I gave him the details, which made me wonder if I'd been hiding my symptoms as well as I thought I'd been. He nodded thoughtfully. "Sorry to hear that," he said and then paused. "Can I ask you a question?"

"Sure."

"What's your biggest fear?"

"That I'll end up in a wheelchair."

"That's good," he said.

"Good?"

"Yup," he said, taking my hand across the table. "That way, you'll never be able to run away from me."

I knew at that moment I'd found the man I wanted to spend the rest of my life with. Eight weeks later, Doug and I were engaged.

THE MYSTERY DEEPENS

Our wedding was June 14, 1997. We honeymooned at sea on a cruise to the Caribbean. Upon returning home, we immediately faced challenges: both of us were laid off from our jobs due to corporate buyouts, and Doug's mother in Sacramento was facing medical issues that made our being closer ideal. Thanks to stock options and severance pay, we were able to do the right thing for us and our family at that time and head north.

Before we left Southern California, however, I had one more important appointment to keep: a visit to Dr. van den Noort. By now, we knew each other well. During my periodic visits, we'd gossip about the hospital business. We'd discuss our shared Dutch heritage and chuckle at our strange-sounding surnames. Despite, or perhaps because of, his gravitas, I called him "Stan the Man," which always made him laugh. "That's Musial," he'd say, referring to the great baseball player who went by the same moniker. "But I'll take it!"

On this visit, however, Stan seemed perplexed.

"Jamie, I'm changing my diagnosis," he said.

"What do you mean?"

"I no longer think you have MS."

"What?"

He held up my most recent MRIs and showed me that after nearly a decade, none of the white plaque lesions that are a hallmark of the disease had yet appeared in my brain.

"If you had MS," he said, pointing to my cerebellum on the MRI, "there'd be white scars here."

"That's great, Stan, I think. But you know I still have the other symptoms?"

He nodded. "I know."

"So if it's not MS, what is it?"

He shook his head. "I wish I could give you an answer. But I'm not sure."

He knew someone who might. A neurologist at UC-Davis, just west of Sacramento. He encouraged me to see him once I'd relocated.

Doug and I had bought a house in a quiet, beautiful neighborhood of the California state capital. Once we settled in, Doug took over the caregiving for his mom, while I found a job in sales, this time for a manufacturer of dictation machines rather than medical sales. But soon after the move, my condition worsened. My legs were getting weaker. Even climbing up a flight of stairs was becoming difficult. I had the so-called "drunken sailor" gait so common to ataxia. There were other complications. At one point, I had problems articulating spoken words and even swallowing.

The specialist at UC-Davis had consulted with Dr. van den Noort. He knew my history and then ran an exhaustive series of tests of his own. The blood work indicated some kind of dysfunction or issues with the mitochondria. Those, students of high school biology will remember, are often referred to as the factories or powerhouses of the cells. So this condition of mine was at the cellular level. What did that mean? What caused it, and more importantly, what could be done to cure it or prevent it from worsening?

It was all so vague. I'd lived for years with the idea of having MS. Oddly, I now felt unanchored in the absence of that diagnosis, as if MS had become part of my identity, like my red hair. Now that was gone, but the weakness, the instability, the vertigo, the blurry vision remained.

The symptoms normally waned and flared, but after a sales-training meeting in San Antonio, they exploded. I had to change planes in Dallas and was trying to catch a connecting flight to Sacramento. There were only minutes to spare, and the next flight wasn't for hours. Pulling my rolling suitcase, I hobbled through the airport trying to get to the gate for the flight to Sacramento. I should have asked for a wheelchair, but I was too proud. *I'm too young to be in a wheelchair in an airport!* I thought.

My gait was off, my legs felt weak, and one eye was getting blurry. As I turned the corridor to my gate, I saw the plane taxiing out on to the runway. I had missed my flight because I was too slow and too proud. Or was it really because my condition was getting significantly worse? I had for years talked about the day that I might be unable to walk. MS or not, was that day now imminent?

I called Doug, crying. "I missed my flight, and I just want to be home with you. I can barely walk. I can't do anything. I feel like I'm falling apart."

Doug, as always, was calm. "Take a deep breath. Then go have dinner, try to relax, and catch the later plane. We'll talk about it when you get home."

I ate dinner, then caught the next flight.

The next day, after Doug arrived home from work, we went out into the backyard and sat in the Jacuzzi. It was a soft, summer night. All very California.

"I felt so bad for you in the airport," he said. "I know it's hard managing your job while you're dealing with whatever this is."

I nodded.

"Maybe you need a break from all that. I think it's time you quit work."

Quit my job? I'd been working my whole life. I was proud of what I'd done in *two* careers, as a nurse and as a sales and marketing professional. Quitting would almost be an admission that this awful illness had won—that it had beaten me and forced me to do something I really didn't want to do. At least not at that point.

One more bout of vertigo, though, was all it took. I realized Doug was right. At just about that time, he got an offer from one of the largest and most prestigious hospital systems in Southern California. Someone high up in the organization knew him and wondered if he might like to return to San Diego and hospital administration. Doug's mother had stabilized, and outside help could be brought in to care for her. The timing seemed right.

Somewhat reluctantly, I agreed. From now on I had to direct my energies on recovering from whatever this "cellular" illness was.

"Maybe we can find a good mitochondria repair guy in San Diego," I said.

"Good idea," deadpanned Doug. "See if you can get him to do an oil change and check the tires while he's at it."

In early 2000, we moved back to San Diego. We found a house in the Scripps Ranch area, and while we didn't think too much about the fact that it was a two-story house at first, soon every step became more labored for me. It quickly became apparent we had made a mistake.

"We're going to have to find a single-level home," Doug said.

I was so upset. The boxes were barely unpacked, and already we had to relocate because of my stupid, malfunctioning mitochondria, or whatever it was.

My walking continued to worsen. I must have been painful to watch, each step slow and draggy. It seemed some days that I had to summon up every ounce of energy and will in order for my legs to shuffle ahead, even just a few inches.

I returned to Dr. van den Noort, and he wrote me a prescription for a scooter. It was humiliating at first, but I had little choice. Doug and I tried to make the most of my new mode of transportation. We'd pop Max, our Pekingese, in the basket of the scooter and I'd race my husband around the block. We laughed, but there really was nothing funny about a forty-year-old woman being forced to use a means of conveyance generally favored by nonagenarians.

One afternoon while Doug was still at work, I sat in the backyard pondering the mysterious condition that had taken over my life. In the past, its symptoms would come and go. There would be a flare-up and then a return to something resembling normal. That day, I realized there was no more normal. My symptoms had been getting worse for months. They would intensify and recede only slightly. My life—our lives—were being turned inside out by whatever was going on inside me. My illness was dictating where we lived. I could no longer work, and now it seemed I could no longer walk.

I tried to hold back tears as I faced the inevitable question: Was I ever going to get better?

CHAPTER 2

The Devastating News

D o you believe in miracles?

After decades working in the medical industry, and as a patient and an advocate, I can't really answer that question with an unequivocal yes. I've seen way too many so-called miracle cures, based on scant or no scientific evidence and designed primarily to get desperate people to pay large amounts of money.

That said, I am a believer, and there's no doubt in my mind that after Doug and I moved to a single-story home in the little town of Ramona, located in the foothills of the Laguna Mountains an hour northeast of San Diego, something miraculous happened to me.

I started to get better.

After fifteen years of battling a mysterious disease that had been diagnosed as various things—MS, a specific form of ataxia, malfunctioning mitochondria, or my favorite, "I'm not sure"—the symptoms slowly but most certainly began to disappear.

According to my internist, the reason for the improvement was that I no longer had to climb stairs and that, having stopped working, I was able to rest when I needed to. Those are probably key factors, but while

I have no studies to prove it, I think another important factor was my change of scenery and the fact that I approached our new living situation with an attitude as clear and fresh as the mountain air.

"Hello, Ramona!" I said aloud one morning after we'd unpacked. "I'm here!"

Aside from the chirping of a few cicadas, Ramona didn't respond.

Why should it? After all, Doug and I certainly were not the first people to be attracted to its idyllic beauty.

———————

To a girl who grew up in a middle-class suburb that was part of a sprawling metropolitan area and then spent most of her life in cities, Ramona was a revelation. Its slow, friendly folkways evoked its cowboy past, a legacy the town manages to accommodate well in the present. It is evidenced by the local Starbucks, one of the few in the country that actually has a hitching post to accommodate horseback drive-throughs.

Located about a mile from the main drag, our house stands atop a hill at the end of a two-hundred-foot driveway. We coexist more or less peaceably with the wildlife and periodic wildfires of the nearby Cleveland National Forest, the edges of which creep down to my backyard, along with the occasional mountain lion and rattlesnake.

After we first arrived, I would gaze out on the valley from our patio at night, illuminated by the light of a thousand stars twinkling in the clear mountain air. That view alone may have done more to restore my spirits, as well as my body, than anything any physician could prescribe.

Doug and I had customized the house for someone with mobility impairment and ever-weakening muscles: no stairs, a walk-in shower, French instead of sliding doors, and—with an eye toward a grim future—a guest suite with its own bathroom for what we both initially expected would be a full-time caregiver for me.

To this point, I'm happy to say, it's been only family and friends who've stayed in that suite, and I'm working hard to keep it that way!

For the first few months after we moved in, I'd still use the scooter outside the house. To accommodate it, we widened an existing footpath that meandered around the property.

Because I was still convinced that my condition would eventually be diagnosed as MS, that's what we told some of the neighbors around us. They were just wonderful. One of them, the vice president of circulation for the *San Diego Union-Tribune*, arranged for our daily newspaper to be dropped off not at the head of the driveway but all the way up by my front door. It was a small but kind gesture, typical of many we got from our Ramona neighbors.

The improvements in my health snuck up on me. One morning in 2003 when I woke up and got out of bed, instead of the first painful, wobbly steps I usually braced for, I was able to walk into the kitchen easily, without looking like a drunken sailor or feeling as if I had ten-pound ankle weights tied around each leg. When I got to the kitchen counter, I realized for once that I wasn't leaning on it for support.

"Oh thank you, God," I said to myself. "I actually feel good."

While that may sound pathetic to someone who has never had what appeared to be a degenerative disease or musculoskeletal injuries, believe me, it was a revelation. I was less fatigued too. Most days I would have been ready for a nap by eleven a.m. Not now. I had been working in our courtyard garden all afternoon the previous day, something that would have normally knocked me out at best, and at worst caused a relapse of vertigo.

That morning I also realized I hadn't used the scooter in, what? Days? Weeks? With a little trepidation, I decided to make a bold gesture. I wheeled it into the garage where, for the most part, it has stayed ever since; a golden-colored reminder of a long, strange period of my life.

That evening, I got the courage to articulate to my husband what I'd been feeling all day.

"Doug, you know what?"

"What?"

"I think . . . I think I'm better."

"Better? As in, *better?*"

"Yeah."

I told him how I'd felt that morning and the changes I'd noticed.

"I think I can finally get around on my own again," I concluded.

"Good," he said, deadpan. "Then you can take out the garbage tonight."

I laughed before he gave me a big hug.

That night I felt normal. Not the new normal, but like the Jamie I remembered back in my twenties. It was so long, I'd almost forgotten what and who that felt like.

BOMBSHELL

I wanted to get back to work, but my internist, who I'd been referred to by Dr. van den Noort, put up a stop sign.

"There are a couple good reasons why you're feeling better," he reminded me. "The fact that you can rest when you need to, and you don't have the stress of a job. So I wouldn't recommend going back to work."

Reluctantly, I admitted he was right. Taking breaks during the day was helpful and likely contributed to my improved sense of well-being. And I probably wasn't ready for the stress of an hour-long commute and a management job that might keep me up worrying at night. But I needed to feel productive, and I could only do so many hours a day in the garden. I began volunteering with local organizations, which was satisfying. But in the back of my mind, I was also perplexed by what had happened to me. Was the previous decade and a half a mirage? Where did that condition and all its terrible symptoms come from? And how was it that even top researchers and diagnosticians like Dr. van den Noort or the neurologist at UC-Davis couldn't come up with a definitive diagnosis?

What seemed like the perfect solution to getting to the bottom of this mystery presented itself in the form of an e-mail I received in late 2008.

It was from a large hospital system in California, inviting me to participate in a research study. "You can help us make a difference," they said. According to the e-mail, they were investigating a simple but important question: If you knew that you had a genetic risk toward certain diseases, would you change your lifestyle to help prevent them?

In other words, if you knew you had a higher than average risk of getting, say, a certain form of cancer, and the evidence suggested that modifying your diet or exercise habits had been shown to lower that risk, would you do it?

The question had currency in 2009, as genetic profiling tests were just then becoming common, most visibly through websites like 23andMe.

The emergence of these new tests had sparked a debate in medical and scientific circles that still continues. Some argued that providing this type of genetic "report card" would result in better lifestyle choices by consumers, including compliance with medical screenings and checkups. Others believed that presenting people with this kind of information would serve only to raise anxiety and perhaps lead them to make rash decisions and undergo unnecessary screenings or procedures.

To participate in the study, I'd need to fill out a detailed family history and then provide saliva in order to have a genetic workup. I would then get to see my risk factors related to a long list of common diseases, which I noticed included MS.

That got my attention.

I agreed to participate in the study. Although these at-home genetic tests were still relatively new at the time, the concept seemed clear. As one news story I read later described such testing, "It's simple: order, spit, ship, and wait."

A few days later a package arrived, containing an eight-inch-long plastic tube with a cap on it. I took the cap off, spit a couple of times into the tube, put the cap back on it, and dropped it off at a local lab that was analyzing the results for the study. Then I sat down to answer the family history online. Although much of it I knew, it still took me two hours and a call to my mom to double-check a few things I was fuzzy on. The questions were about my parents and siblings: How old were they? If deceased, at what age and what was the cause of death? If they were alive, did they have health issues?

My siblings were fine. But my dad, then in his midseventies, had been diagnosed with Alzheimer's disease the previous year. It was so upsetting that I'd tried to put it in the back of my mind.

"Why are you doing this?" Doug asked as he saw me laboring over the questionnaire. "Are you concerned about a genetic risk for something?"

I told him that in return for providing the family history and saliva sample, participants would receive a detailed breakdown of their genetic risk for about twenty different diseases, including MS.

"This is my chance to find out if I really had it," I said.

"But you're doing so much better," he said. "And the MRIs on your brain were negative, right?"

"Right, but I still want to know."

It was hard to explain, even to Doug, but there was a part of me that couldn't accept maybe for an answer. I needed some closure on the nature of the affliction I'd battled for so many years. And although I certainly was doing a lot better, there were times my legs still didn't feel quite right, and who was to say these symptoms wouldn't come back? I felt all along that Dr. van den Noort's original diagnosis had been correct. Maybe I was that rare MS patient who didn't have lesions on the brain. Who knows? But certainly, having a genetic predisposition to that disease would help answer the question conclusively.

"Up to you, obviously," Doug said, when I'd explained my somewhat dubious reasoning. "I'm not sure if I'd want to know my risks for all these things."

That, as I have learned in subsequent years, is not an atypical attitude. A lot of people don't want to know. But I did. I finished the questionnaire, hit Send, and waited for my results.

They arrived in April 2009, in an e-mail with a twenty-nine-page PDF attachment. I went scrolling through to find what I was looking for: a summary page entitled "Your Estimated Lifetime Risk."

There, arrayed in neat columns, was a list of common diseases, with two percentages next to each: the subject's risk of getting the disease, compared to the average of the population.

I perused the list, noting that my odds of getting Lupus, Crohn's disease, or atrial fibrillations were considerably lower than average. Good to know. Then I found what I was looking for: multiple sclerosis. Now we're going to get to the bottom of this!

But I felt myself quickly deflating as I read that the average estimated lifetime risk for contracting MS was .77 percent. Mine was only .36. I had a lower than average risk for the disease that I thought had been afflicting me for most of my adult life! So much for my theory. While it didn't conclusively answer the question of what I'd suffered from, there was clearly no genetic predisposition toward MS.

What a waste of time.

And then on the top right-hand side of the page, I noticed my scores for Alzheimer's disease:

Average: 17 percent

You: 75 percent

I gasped. "What? Alzheimer's?"

I clicked through for more information.

You have 2 of the 2 risk markers we looked for.

Those words were like a flashlight shining on my face in a dark alley. "That's her," says the voice of the genetic police. "She's the one that's got what we've been looking for."

But what exactly *were* they looking for? *What do I have?*

It turns out the gene they were looking for is ApoE4. And to make matters worse, I didn't have just one of these genes but two.

I searched the rest of the report in hopes that maybe I'd find some kind of large asterisk or disclaimer. Maybe I'd get an e-mail of apology saying I'd gotten someone else's report by accident. But no, it was mine, all mine. And my further research that evening only made this realization worse. I googled this ApoE gene, and on the National Institute on Aging website I found a description: "ApoE4 increases risk for Alzheimer's disease and is also associated with an earlier age of disease onset."[1]

I was shattered.

But the NIA entry went on to say that inheriting this variation of the gene did not mean that a person will *definitely* develop Alzheimer's. A ray of hope? I tried to calm myself, taking a deep breath and telling myself maybe it wasn't as bad as I thought. But then I noticed that they kept referring to "an" ApoE4 gene. As in one. According to my genetic profile results, I had inherited two, a genetic gift from both sides of the family.

More googling, and finally I found a Duke University paper, which reported that those individuals like me unlucky enough to have two of these genes actually had a 91 percent lifetime risk of getting Alzheimer's disease. I later learned the average onset age was sixty-three to sixty-five.

Ninety one percent. And it would happen at an age when most people are just getting ready to retire and enjoy their lives.

Long-forgotten memories of Grandma Neva drooling in her wheelchair flashed into my mind.

My medical training as well as my personal medical history had taught me to stay calm and be rational. But I wasn't ready for this.

I pushed my chair away from the screen and wandered out of my office in a daze.

Doug got home and found me sitting, ashen, on the couch. I was still numb over this news.

"Hi," he said.

I looked up at him. "I just found out I have a 91 percent chance of getting Alzheimer's disease. How was your day?"

Doug's eyes widened momentarily. I explained the test results. "And please don't tell me 'I told you so,'" I concluded. "You were right. I probably shouldn't have done this."

"Nah," Doug said, "it's no big deal."

"What do you mean no big deal? This is like a guarantee that I'm going to get Alzheimer's." I thought about it for a second. "Doug, I'm worried you're going to have to take care of me."

"That's what you're worried about? Well, don't give that a second thought."

"Why not?"

He grinned. "I'm a lot older than you. I'll be dead by the time you get it."

WELCOME TO THE "4/4" CLUB

The next morning, I woke up with a headache. And with every throb, it seemed like "91 percent" was reverberating through my head. I also began to think about my family. I had the memories of Grandma Neva, and I'd seen my mom struggle with my grandmother when she lost her memory near the end of her life. Now my father had recently been diagnosed with Alzheimer's. That's three relatives right there. All this time I'd been focused on the wrong disease. Instead of worrying whether I had MS, I should have been thinking about the fact that I might get Alzheimer's. Why hadn't I considered my family tree and put two and two together?

Two and two equals four. My new unlucky number.

All right, then. It's time to get organized. I booted up the computer and printed out the entire genetic report plus some of the other documents I'd found the previous night and placed them all in a binder. I was going to start learning about this, and I was ready to take action. This study was about whether the knowledge of a genetic predisposition would alter one's behavior, right? *Okay, then, I'm ready to alter my behavior if it will help. I'll exercise more, eat better. I'll even promise to never take a sip of Doug's chardonnay again.* (My husband could be very protective when it came to his favorite wine.) *Tell me what to do. I'm your girl.*

Since I was at high risk for the disease, my genetic report had included a couple of pages of information on Alzheimer's. While it tried to sound upbeat and included a list of promising studies and boilerplate diet and exercise recommendations, two sentences jumped out at me: "There is no known cure for Alzheimer's" and "As of yet, there are no surefire strategies for preventing Alzheimer's."

No prevention. No treatment. No cure.

I was beginning to feel like I had just been given a genetic death sentence, and there was no way to have it commuted and no time off for good behavior.

Later, as I became lost in despair, I learned that even Doug's attempts at levity had been a bit of a smokescreen too. My wonderful husband, who had always fixed everything for me—getting me the right house to live in, getting me the right scooter—couldn't fix this. A few days after I told him the news, he called our life insurance broker and increased the benefit amount of our policy, presumably in the event I needed a lot of expensive care if he died before me.

At that point, would I even know?

————————

I was one of more than three thousand people who participated in the study, the results of which were later published in a prestigious medical journal. The researchers found that undergoing the genetic testing did not result in any measurable changes in exercise, diet, or screenings.

Consider me the minority vote, because based on what I'd gleaned from the test—that I had an extremely high predisposition toward Alzheimer's disease—I was ready to do all of the above recommendations and more!

But first I needed to better understand the study and the science behind it.

I decided to contact the principal investigator (PI), Dr. Prescott F. Leyland, a prominent physician and researcher. I wrote him an e-mail that, in part, read:

> Dear Dr. Leyland:
>
> I volunteered to be a participant in your genome study. I have been informed that I have two copies of the ApoE4 gene, which puts me at a very high risk for Alzheimer's disease, and I am a bit anxious. I thought that knowing this information would be helpful. Unfortunately, there exists a great divide between acquiring this knowledge and what to do with it.

As an RN, I thought he might be willing to talk to me, explain a little bit more about the thinking behind the study and what my results meant. Perhaps he'd give me a verbal hug and a referral to a neurologist for a consult.

I heard nothing. After resending the e-mail and cc'ing Dr. Leyland's CEO, I heard back from his assistant, who scheduled a meeting.

I arrived around ten a.m. at his large, plush suite of offices. I opened the door and found a TV crew set up in the lobby. There were lights, cameras, technicians, a sound man, and a crisply suited, hair-perfectly-coiffed TV reporter standing with the white-coated Dr. Leyland.

They appeared to be wrapping up.

I could see this guy must be important. He had the local news there doing a story about him. The crew began to pack up. I made my way through the crowd and identified myself to the receptionist.

"Oh, right," she said, looking at his schedule. "Okay, hold on."

Dr. Leyland was still chatting amicably with the reporter when I saw her go over to him and whisper in his ear. I saw an almost imperceptible look of annoyance sweep across his face before he turned back and apologized to the reporter. "I'm sorry, I have to take care of something," he said, smiling and obsequious. "Thank you so much for coming down to talk to us. Your questions were really good."

He then strode past me and back through the reception door into the offices inside.

A few minutes later, I was summoned. Instead of his office, I was ushered into a conference room, where he sat looking at his phone. It was a cold, sterile room with a wooden table. He sat on the opposite end.

"Let me just finish sending this," he said briskly, tapping a few more keystrokes. "Okay," he said and looked up. "So you are—?"

"Jamie. Jamie Tyrone."

"Right. So how can I help you?"

"I was a participant in your genetic disease risk study."

"Yes, right, I remember your e-mail now. It's been a hectic day here, as you can see." He looked at me, drumming his fingers. I gathered that was my cue to state my business and make it snappy.

"Thank you for seeing me, doctor," I said. I reminded him of the findings. "I'm having some anxiety about the information I got in the study."

"We take pride in doing good research here, you know," he said, as if I'd just questioned his abilities.

I was taken aback and started to say something about how I had no doubt as to the quality of his research. Indeed, I was aware that this particular study had been partially funded by the National Institutes of Health. But he went on talking. "We have several other people who found they were at risk for various diseases, and they weren't upset. You should be happy."

Happy? That I've got a 91 percent chance of getting Alzheimer's? I felt my face flush.

"Now you can change your lifestyle to help prevent it. You can eat better, decrease your cholesterol, and start exercising more."

This was basically a rehash of everything that was in the boilerplate of the results. Clearly, I wasn't going to get any new information from him. And he didn't look like the kind of guy who gave hugs, verbal or otherwise.

"Okay, well thanks," I said, reigning in my frustration. "Last question. Can you refer me to a neurologist so I can follow up with this? Or maybe even an Alzheimer's researcher? I'd like to learn a little bit more about this."

"No, I'm sorry I can't," he said. "I don't really know any neurologists. Or anybody who does work in Alzheimer's."

He then extended his hand, indicating our meeting was over.

"Boy, he wasn't very nice," I told Doug that night. "He couldn't get me out of his office fast enough."

"He was probably just freaked out that you showed up," Doug said.

"A little bit, I think. But still, that doesn't excuse his behavior toward me. What about some compassion?"

"You're right," he said, "but I think you've got two roads you can take here with this whole situation. The high road or the low road. I hope you choose the right one."

The next day, I took my first steps on what I thought would be the high road. I called the local Alzheimer's Association office, explained my situation, and asked if they had any support groups for those who had my same genetic risk.

"APO what?" said the kindly man who answered the phone. "I'm sorry, I don't think I know what that is. But we do have a lot of support groups here, and we'd love to try and help you."

I thanked him and hung up. Then I thought back to my sales days and had an idea. Sometimes, when you're rejected, the right approach is to come back to the prospective client with a different offer. I sat down and composed an e-mail to Dr. Leyland.

I knew his hospital had a department of integrative medicine— basically a patient-centered area of medicine that looks for interdisciplinary solutions to health problems. If he could put me in touch with someone in that area, I proposed working together to develop a brain health program.

I was trying to show him how reasonable I could be. And that maybe we could work collaboratively. He was receptive. This time he managed to come up with a name.

The high road was getting me places.

But the department chair for integrative medicine wouldn't even talk to me. "She's busy for the next six months on another project," her assistant told me.

Six months? She couldn't take even five minutes to speak?

I went back to Dr. Leyland, thanked him again for being supportive of my idea. But could he possibly nudge the department chair or give me another name? An e-mail from him would certainly open doors.

The response I received left me cold: "I've done enough for you. Please don't call me again."

I had never received an e-mail like this, even as a sales rep.

I was not being taken seriously. I was not being listened to. I was hurt and alone. I was being ignored. And I had questions, but no one seemed interested enough to answer.

One thing I yearned to know was, why wasn't any genetic counseling provided? I had been reading up on the guidelines for genetic testing, and I should have been assigned a counselor for at least a phone consultation during the consent process and before the consultation. Instead, this earth-shattering news was just e-mailed to me.

Finally, after numerous e-mails to various people at the hospital, I got the answer: too expensive.

I was furious. And I was now getting desperate. I suppose you could say I had been living in what we might call "healthy denial." As I thought about my three relatives who had Alzheimer's or senility, sure, maybe it made sense. But I hadn't thought about it, and I had no symptoms.

Now, I started to imagine symptoms every day. I'd worry every time I couldn't find a word. Every time I misplaced my car keys. Every time I forgot the name of a movie or a book. Before 2009, I wouldn't have thought twice about any of that. But now I had this strange sequence of letters and numbers etched into my brain—ApoE4 times two, or "4/4"—every moment of forgetfulness left me terrified.

Could this be it?

That's when I went into a tailspin. For about three months, I wouldn't get out of bed. I didn't clean the house or tend to the garden. And when

Doug finally came home, all I would do was carp about Alzheimer's, Dr. Leyland, and the study.

One night he said to me, "I don't know how long I can continue living with you like this." Even Doug, my unwavering supporter, was getting sick of my behavior. My questions grew darker. Do I really want to be here anymore? What do I have to look forward to? A wheelchair and drool? I had a bottle of Benadryl in our medicine cabinet. Some Vicodin, too, for pain relief. Thoughts of downing a bottle of Vicodin along with a bottle of liquor filled my head. Then I'd never have to worry about Alzheimer's again.

I was thinking seriously about when and where to do it. But a couple of things stopped me.

First, a brush with faith. I had been raised Lutheran, but at one point in my adult life I had attended a Catholic church as part of my spiritual searching. I remembered learning why suicide was considered a mortal sin to Catholics. The preservation of life, body and soul, was not something discretionary, I had read. It was an obligation you owed to yourself, your family, and to God. "We are stewards, not owners, of the life God has entrusted to us. It is not ours to dispose"—that was the line I remembered in the catechism.

Although no longer a practicing Catholic, I still found those words stirring. And thinking about them at the lowest point during my crisis made me second-guess my morbid plan. As did the whole idea of walking away from this problem. Okay, so maybe I was destined to get Alzheimer's. But I had never stepped down from a challenge. I'd gotten back on the horse in nursing school after my patient's tragic death on my first day in the hospital. I'd stood up to a couple of haughty OR physicians as a young RN. I'd persevered despite my disabling and mysterious illness of the previous decades, and now I could walk like a human being again.

I'd faced all those situations. There were things I could do here too.

I was sure of it. And not just the lifestyle modifications that I knew were important. Maybe I could help in other ways so that, if not me, others might not have to live with this kind of genetic sword hanging over their heads.

That hope was realized when, out of the blue, a woman at the testing company contacted me. Jenny was one of the few associated with the study who had shown any interest in helping me. She called to tell me that she had spoken to a Dr. Eric Reiman at the Banner Alzheimer's Institute (BAI) in Arizona. Jenny told me that Banner was a top-notch research facility and that she'd explained to Dr. Reiman about my test results and indicated my interest in learning more and perhaps in getting active in research or advocacy.

"He said he'd be happy to speak to you, Jamie," she said. "I think he might be the guy you're looking for."

Jenny had gone above and beyond, and I will always be grateful to her for connecting me with Dr. Reiman. Several years later I met her face-to-face for the first time at a conference. "Thank you so much for that referral, Jenny," I said. "You were really kind to do that."

"It was the least I could do," she responded. Her eyes hardened. "I have to tell you, I wish I'd never been affiliated with that study."

"Well," I said, "that makes two of us."

Looking back, I realize this sudden prospect of a life with Alzheimer's managed to distract me from the ongoing puzzle of life with what had appeared to be MS. While the symptoms lessened, to this day I can't help but wonder if there was some kind of connection behind whatever that elusive affliction was and my ApoE 4/4 status.

Regardless, I now had a new and even more daunting fight on my hands.

CHAPTER 3

Adventures of a Lab Rat

D r. Reiman seemed to know all about my genetic status, my frustrating interactions with Dr. Leyland, the lack of genetic counseling made available to me, how my efforts to start a brain health program had been rebuffed, and, I'm sure, my various meltdowns over the whole thing.

"You went through an unfortunate experience," he said. "I'm sorry."

Right away he validated my feeling that the situation had been mishandled. Finally, someone was listening.

Besides being a compassionate person, Dr. Reiman is a highly respected researcher and the executive director of the Banner Alzheimer's Institute. He is also the author of more than four hundred publications and received the prestigious Potamkin Prize, which essentially is a Nobel or Pulitzer Prize for research on Alzheimer's disease.

Dr. Reiman knew full well what it meant to be a "4/4"—shorthand for someone like me who had two sets of the ApoE4 gene—and explained more to me about the genetic structure I'd inherited. "Yes, you're at high risk," he said. "But remember, that's not a guarantee you're going to get it."

I appreciated his positivity but politely told him that while I'm not much of a gambler, if I were in Vegas and someone told me I had a 91 percent chance of winning at craps, I'd be at the table with a pair of dice in my hand.

He laughed. "I hear what you're saying, but did you know there are people in their eighties who are 4/4, don't have Alzheimer's, and are cognitively normal? There might be other genes or mechanisms that we don't yet understand that could be at play here, mitigating the risk posed by having both of those genes."

I nodded thoughtfully. "That's good to hear," I said, "but in the meantime, I'd like to be able to do something. I was wondering, is there any way I could be a participant in one of your studies?"

Even though I was too young for much of the research on Alzheimer's, Dr. Reiman thought it was a capital idea and told me about some investigations that were currently underway at Banner. One in particular was a longitudinal (long-term) study being done in conjunction with the Mayo Clinic in which biomarkers—such as plaques in the brain and the volume of the hippocampus, the memory center of the brain, and cognitive abilities, as well as genetic status—would be followed and tested over time.

"That sounds fascinating," I said. "I'd love to be part of it."

Because this was a long-term Alzheimer's study and subjects as young as forty-nine could be admitted, I met the criteria. But honestly, I couldn't help wonder if part of the reason Dr. Reiman invited me to participate is that he wanted me to see that not all researchers were cold and dispassionate. If so, he succeeded. Working with him and his colleagues at Banner was a revelation. From that very first phone conversation, I was allowed to ask questions and not get dismissive answers. And boy, did I get some answers. I learned more about Alzheimer's in general and my particular condition in ten minutes with Eric than I had in ten months of googling.

"Great," he said, when I agreed to be part of the study. "I'll have my research coordinator contact you to work out the details."

A few months later, I arrived in Phoenix for three days of testing at the Banner Alzheimer's Institute. Dr. Reiman himself was there to meet me the morning I walked in. A gentle bear of a man with a warm smile and a serene presence, he immediately put me at ease. "Welcome to Banner, Jamie," he said.

First, I was ushered through a series of tests: MRI, PET scan, blood work. Everyone made me feel special; like I was already a valuable contributor to the important work going on there, and I'd barely walked in the door! Of course, the real rock stars at Banner were the researchers. They had produced groundbreaking papers there. In fact, although I didn't meet him at the time, I learned that one of the institute's big names was a neurologist who enters our story soon: Dr. Marwan Sabbagh, the coauthor of this book.

When we broke for lunch that first day, Banner had thoughtfully provided food, a healthy salad. Then it was on to cognitive testing, which was conducted by Dr. Richard Casselli from the Mayo Clinic. "Your lab rat is here!" I announced, throwing my arms up theatrically. Dr. Casselli looked aghast.

"We don't like that term," he said. "You're a 'research partner.'"

"Whatever you say, Doctor Casselli, I'm just happy to be part of the study. But I have to warn you, I already ate the lab rat salad, with extra cheese."

He smiled sweetly, although I suspect what he was thinking was "Oh boy, just what I need—a research subject who's a comedian."

The reason I was trying to lighten the mood was that I was nervous. I think people equate cognitive testing with an examination of one's intelligence. I was expecting them to test my knowledge. (*If they ask me the main characters in* War and Peace *or to name the presidents in order,*

I thought, *I'm sunk!*) But it wasn't like *Jeopardy* or Trivial Pursuit, or, thankfully, the SATs.

In fact, the first part of the neurocognitive test was more physical. Dr. Casselli had me stand on one leg at a time, with eyes closed and arms raised, to check my balance. He had me walk back and forth in "tandem" fashion, with one foot in front of the other, to assess my gait. He asked me to follow his fingers—side to side, close up, and back—as he observed the way my eyes tracked his movements.

Then a neuropsychologist took over the exam. He showed me a series of shapes and images to see if I could recognize and distinguish among them. For example, he would flash a protractor and a ruler and ask if I could tell the difference. At one point in the test I panicked, because I couldn't immediately recognize a yoke—the crosspiece typically used with teams of oxen. I had some big laughs with some of the staff about that later. "Come on, that's not fair," I said. "I grew up in the LA suburbs! What do I know about farming equipment?"

Much more testing was to come, but all kidding aside, for those three days at Banner, I finally felt as if I was making a difference. It wouldn't be immediate—in fact, the study is still ongoing—but I allowed myself to believe that I'd done my small part in the long campaign to eventually alter that bleak no-prevention, no-treatment, no-cure Alzheimer's prognosis.

Personally, I felt I'd also taken a step out of my morass of despair.

My good feelings didn't last though. After I returned home, I read an article about a new study, not done at Banner, suggesting that the amyloid plaque that is a key marker of Alzheimer's can begin forming as much as twenty years before onset of the disease.

I did a quick mental calculation. If average onset for someone with my genetic risk was in their midsixties, that meant plaque could be growing inside my head now. The idea of that horrified and tortured me. I had nightmares of wormlike lesions slithering through my brain. Every time I had a routine memory lapse, I imagined these plaques crushing some vital part of my brain as they grew like kudzu.

Hysterical, I called Dr. Reiman. I told him what I read. "I could be talking to you right now and these plaques are growing in my brain," I cried.

A board-certified psychiatrist (on top of all of his other credentials), Dr. Reiman doubtless had experience dealing with distraught patients. He reassured me that these lesions, if they were even present, were not gobbling their way through my brain like giant earthworms in a 1950s horror movie. But he was concerned, because he was about to leave on a trip for Europe for the next two weeks. "I want to make sure you have someone you can call while I'm gone, if you need it," he said. "I'm going to put Dr. Adam Fleischer on 'Jamie duty.'"

Shortly after that call, on August 23, Doug and his family and I were at Newport Beach, celebrating my birthday. I was trying to have fun, but I was still pretty upset. My phone rang. It was a Phoenix number.

"Hello?"

"Hi, Jamie, this is Dr. Adam Fleischer at Banner. Just wanted to check in and see how you're doing."

I was almost moved to tears. "Thank you so much for reaching out to me, doctor. I know you probably think I'm some high maintenance lunatic who—"

"No, no," he interrupted. "We're all very fond of you here. I also know you're eager to learn and get more involved with this, which is why I'm calling."

"Another study?"

"Actually, another institute. You're in San Diego, right? Did you know that UCSD has one of the best Alzheimer's centers in the country? It's been around for decades, and it's right in your backyard!"

I was momentarily flummoxed at the idea that the University of California–San Diego—less than an hour's drive from Ramona—had such an institute. Why did no one involved with the genetic study mention this to me to begin with?

"I hope you don't mind," Adam continued. "I've contacted a colleague of mine there, and she's going to call you."

A few weeks later, I was sitting in the office of Mary Sundsmo, program director for the UCSD Shiley-Marcos Alzheimer's Disease Research Center (ADRC). Despite its long and well-endowed name, there was nothing off-putting about the center—or, for that matter, Mary, who as I always liked to say wrapped her angel wings around me the first time she met me.

"Jamie," she said, giving me a hug. "It's so nice to meet you. Come sit down and let's talk."

We sat down, not at a round table in some sterile conference room, but in two comfortable chairs facing each other in her office. We were separated by a small table upon which had been placed a vase of freshly cut flowers.

In that bright and cheery setting, I did what she had invited me to do: I talked. And talked. And talked. Mary heard my whole story, and I cried as I told her how this whole situation had affected my life and how fragile my psyche had become. I confessed that I was walking around with the numbers 91 percent and 4/4 twirling in my mind, while imagining rapacious lesions growing in my head.

At that point, Dr. Doug Galasko, who was the director of the ADRC at the time, popped his head in. Mary introduced us. "I didn't know 4/4s really existed," she said. Dr. Galasko smiled and nodded toward me. "Yes, they do, and now you're meeting one."

I had learned by that point that only 2 percent of the population had two sets of the ApoE4 gene. At that moment, I felt like a genetic celebrity. The positive embrace by Mary and her colleagues at the ADRC, combined with what I'd experienced at Banner, began the shift for me.

I realized now I had allies in this struggle to regain my life and my sanity—and to find some purpose in it.

"Jamie, you always have a home here," Mary said at the end of our meeting.

Driving back to Ramona, I felt inspired. Instead of bemoaning my fate, I wanted to do something. A first key step was participating in research. But certainly I had skills from my career as a nurse and my years in sales and marketing. Couldn't I put these to use to help the mission of my new friends; the good people at Banner and the ADRC trying to fight the disease I was carrying around in my DNA? I was fired up and ready to go.

Mary recognized this. She began including me in more of the ADRC activities. I attended conferences, meet-and-greets, and meetings. I helped decorate rooms for events, creating floral arrangements. I even offered to stuff envelopes. I was there for whatever she needed. Mary also knew I wanted to learn, so she invited me to sit in when visiting scholars presented the latest research and other topics related to AD. I began to read the studies in order to better understand not just my condition but the disease as a whole, as well as what was being done to combat it.

One day I got a call from Dr. Reiman's office at Banner. He needed to talk to me.

"I hear you're getting involved with our friends at the ADRC," he said. I thanked him and Adam again for referring me.

"Well, Jamie, I know you want to get more involved, and there may be another opportunity for you," he said.

"I'm all ears."

Dr. Reiman explained that he had been contacted by a producer at CNN. They were doing a documentary about Banner's groundbreaking trial in Columbia. Even though the trial was based on a gene mutation, CNN also wanted to interview someone who had a high genetic risk.

"So," I said, "you thought of your favorite 4/4?"

"I certainly did. But Jamie, before you say yes, I really want you to think about it. You realize that this will mean you can no longer be anonymous about your status."

That would be a serious decision. Genetic test results may affect your ability to obtain life, disability, and long-term care insurance.

But I wanted to support Dr. Reiman and Banner. I knew there were other people out there with similar backgrounds, if not quite the same genetic structure. Perhaps learning about me would help reassure them that they aren't alone. Perhaps it would also encourage research participation.

"Thanks, Doctor Reiman," I said, "but you know what? I'm ready to go public."

The documentary, *Filling the Blanks*, aired on CNN in January 2011, and later won an award.

I was happy to see that Dr. Reiman was interviewed extensively for the show, as were other prominent researchers whose names I recognized. Much of it was filmed in a remote area of Colombia, where there is a cluster of families with a rare genetic mutation that leads to a frighteningly high incidence of early onset AD. My segment entailed a crew coming to my home to film me in front of my computer, and then following me for a visit with my dad, also diagnosed with AD. Dad mugged for the camera a bit and actually looked pretty dapper with his white handlebar mustache, although the segment captures on film the fact that while he recognized me, he couldn't remember my name.

For the most part, Dad was able to put up a good front that day. But six months after the documentary aired, he died.

When I saw the finished piece, I was shaken by some of the stories of others. I saw that I wasn't the only one who had been traumatized by the knowledge that they had a genetic risk for AD. I saw the suffering of patients and the heartache and bravery of caregivers.

"We have a lot of work to do," I declared on camera, near the end of the documentary.

Now becoming clear that my work was as an advocate, I plunged myself into the fight while I continued to work out my own complex and volatile emotions concerning my genetic status.

A few years later, Mary invited me to speak at the ADRC's thirtieth anniversary celebration. The University of California–San Diego has a long, storied history in Alzheimer's research. In fact, it's not an overexaggeration to say that a lot of serious research into AD began here. An audience of about 150 had gathered at a posh local country club to mark the occasion, and Mary asked me to be the final speaker, to share with the audience what the ADRC meant to me.

I was nervous, but I had written what I thought was a concise and impactful speech. I asked the audience essentially to put themselves in my shoes, emphasizing the word *imagine*:

> *Imagine* knowing that you inherited two copies of a gene, one from each parent, which puts you at a 91 percent lifetime risk of succumbing to Alzheimer's disease.
>
> *Imagine* fearing that you will become the next burden to a loving family.
>
> *Imagine* looking into your father's empty eyes and realizing that you are looking into a mirror that reflects your own destiny.
>
> I can't imagine this, because this is my reality. I am that person.
>
> Approximately six years ago, I was told of my genetic status . . . I was not given any information or support as to how to deal with this information.
>
> After trying to navigate this journey alone, a miracle happened! This miracle gave me a home to feel safe in. A home full of support and love all wrapped up with a big hug. That home is the Shiley-Marcos Alzheimer's Disease Research Center. And because of their

collaborative efforts with other research centers, I was given one of the greatest purposes in life, and that was becoming a "lab rat" for research. It is because of the Shiley-Marcos ADRC that I am able to fulfill what I see as my obligation to make sense of this information and to make a difference in the fight against this disease. It is because of the support of wonderful people like you that I am able to fulfill my purpose and help find a cure. It is because of the wonderful support of the ADRC that I am on the road to healing.

That night, a reporter from the *Union-Tribune* was in the audience. She was impressed enough to call Mary, who connected us. The reporter, Michele Parente, ended up writing a profile on me. What would I call myself, I wondered, if I were writing the headline for that story? An Alzheimer's time bomb? Someone who had come out of the genetic closet? A loser in the 4/4 lottery? Of course, that's not how it ended up in Michele's piece. "Living with a 91 Percent Chance of Alzheimer's" was the headline, but I was grateful for the front-page story, not to mention the many e-mails and calls I got as a result. I decided that continuing to share my experience as honestly as I could might be beneficial to others.

When I got another request from Banner to participate in a panel discussion in Phoenix, I eagerly accepted. As usual, it was me, the 4/4 freak, with a group of experts speaking to a lay audience, most of whom were probably either dealing with AD or alarmed at the prospect. When I was introduced, I told my tale of genetic woe and the initial lack of support.

As I concluded, the panelist next to me put his hand over the microphone in order to share a private exchange of words. I knew him, a distinguished researcher in AD.

"Jamie," he said, "I'm so sorry."

I was touched by the reaction of this handsome, dark-haired man. Not that he could have helped alter my genetic fate. Nor did he have anything to do with the original study, the treatment I received, or the anxiety it had caused. And yet he, a prominent researcher in AD, whose name I recognized from reading journal articles and books, still wanted to express his concern. "Thank you, doctor," I said. "That's really kind of you. I appreciate it."

He smiled and continued in a whisper. "We were introduced to the audience, but I don't think you and I have officially met," he said, smiling and extending his hand. "I'm Marwan. Marwan Sabbagh."

CHAPTER 4

The ABCs of ALZ

MARWAN SABBAGH, MD

I was impressed by Jamie's story. While she was not the first person I'd met with the 4/4 genetic risk, it's highly unusual, and I admired her courage and honesty in standing up in front of an audience to tell her story.

Sadly, what she experienced in 2009 is still relevant a decade later. Despite the advances in genetic science and the plethora of personalized information we can now gather, we don't seem to have advanced very far in terms of how that information is communicated. You can still just spit in a tube, pay a modest fee, and seemingly have your genetic future foretold, without any context, without any consultation, without any expert who can help interpret the results.

This is especially true with Alzheimer's disease and its seemingly grim prognosis. That's my specialty.

I grew up in Tucson, Arizona, part of a family of doctors. By the age of eight, I knew that I, too, wanted to be a physician. My dad encouraged me, giving me a copy of *Grey's Anatomy* for my fourteenth birthday. Four years later, at age eighteen, I started doing research in Alzheimer's. As they say, I never looked back. It has been my life's work. I'm often asked why. Why this disease? It's a good question. Alzheimer's doesn't run in my family. Nor does it seem to be the kind of specialty that would have attracted the interest of a young premed college student in the 1980s.

The answer is simple: fear of growing old is what drove me. While for many, aging can be a rich and wonderful experience, AD seems the opposite. It seems to me the embodiment of everything sad and tragic about growing old. Those disturbing memories Jamie has of visiting her great-grandmother are not unique. Granted, the caregiving standards may have changed, and instead of sitting around in fetid hospital dayrooms, patients with AD today engage in often healthy activities at adult day-care centers. Still, as someone who has diagnosed more cases of this disease than I'd care to recall, as someone who has seen its worst effects, how it ravages the body and breaks hearts as well as minds, I can tell you this: Alzheimer's is a disease worth fighting. And I'm proud to have devoted my career to doing that.

And you know what? All that work by so many of us—from the ADRC in San Diego to Banner to Cleveland Clinic—may be finally paying off. Let me be clear on this. After twenty-five years in the field, I've seen a lot of disappointments and dead ends, which is one reason for the no-prevention, no-treatment, no-cure mantra you hear again and again when it comes to AD. For example, we have not had a new drug approved for Alzheimer's since 2003. That's more than fifteen years! I doubt there is any other major disease for which new medications have been lagging for so long. It's a dismal record, admittedly. Some say it's because we're looking at the wrong targets; some say we're treating it too late; some say our methods are wrong.

I say despite that, the future for AD treatment is bright. Exciting new evidence is emerging that comprehensive lifestyle interventions can make a difference. Promising treatments are not just on the horizon but close enough that we may see them introduced in clinical settings soon. And I believe that in the near future we may be able to at last modify the "no cure" label for AD.

Notice that I did not say we will have a cure. That's a word that makes researchers wince. But we have reason to believe that as it happened with some forms of cancer, rheumatoid arthritis, and many other once-hopeless diseases, in the near future we may be able to consider AD a treatable if not curable disease.

That would be a huge change. But you don't have to sit and wait for it to transpire. There are things you can do now, much as Jamie has done. The latest research is a clear call to action. You can engage in preventive strategies, some of which we will detail later. And you can start today. Don't wait until you or a loved one starts showing symptoms. (I have included a list of symptoms later in this chapter.)

First, let's look at the science behind the disease that upended Jamie's life and that, sadly, has destroyed the lives of so many others. But as we do, keep in mind that the picture is a changing one, and there is every reason for optimism in the fight against a disease that we never even knew existed until the early 1900s.

BEGINNINGS

In November 1906, at a meeting of a professional association of German psychiatrists, a dapper, mustachioed man in his early forties rose to give a presentation. He described a "peculiar severe disease process of the cerebral cortex" that he had identified in a recently deceased patient.[1]

The presenter's name was Dr. Alois Alzheimer, and at the time he began studying the brain of Auguste Deter—a fifty-one-year-old woman who had been admitted to the local asylum in Frankfurt—he was already a distinguished psychiatrist and pathologist.

Dr. Alzheimer had followed the progression of Deter's disease for five years. Her symptoms included memory loss, unpredictable behavior, and confusion. Upon her death, he examined her brain under a microscope and discovered two abnormalities: tangles that had formed on the nerve cells and plaque deposits that had emerged between the cells. In his speech, Alzheimer claimed that the patient's dementia was related to these abnormalities.

The good doctor was right on much of what he theorized about the condition that now bears his name. But his findings, as another writer on the history of the disease observed, were met with a collective yawn. The illness Alzheimer had identified was consigned to the back pages of the medical texts and believed to be an anomaly, a rare condition that few physicians would ever see.

One of the key figures in changing that view of Alzheimer's was one of my mentors, Dr. Robert Katzman of the University of California–San Diego, who had looked at the brains of patients with symptoms similar to Deter's and discovered that they had the same characteristics. In 1976, he published a groundbreaking editorial in the journal *Archives of Neurology* entitled "The Prevalence and Malignancy of Alzheimer's Disease." His paper said, in essence, that many if not most of the patients that had been lumped together by the medical community as "senile" actually had the same condition the obscure German psychiatrist had identified seventy years earlier.[2]

Suddenly, the disease went from being very rare to all too common. According to *The New York Times*, prior to the publication of his paper, fewer than 150 scientific articles had been published about the disease. From 1976 until Dr. Katzman's death in 2008, forty-five thousand articles were published. In his obituary, he would be hailed by the *Times* as having redefined the disease as a major public health problem.[3]

As for Alois Alzheimer, his name would become a synonym for an end-of-life existence that some feel is worse than death.

WHAT IS ALZHEIMER'S DISEASE?

If few were listening to Dr. Alzheimer's lecture in 1906, there is enormous interest today in the disease that bears his name. I see it in my own presentations. As a specialist in dementia and Alzheimer's disease, I frequently give lectures across the country to colleagues and students who are working on developing treatments and to people who are interested in the latest research. Typically, the average person wants to know three things:

1. Am I getting Alzheimer's?
2. What is my risk for getting AD?
3. What can I do about it?

I'd like to add a fourth question that is not asked quite as frequently by the lay public but should be:

4. Exactly what is Alzheimer's disease?

I think it's important to understand what the disease is. And it's equally important to recognize what it's not.

Simply stated, Alzheimer's is a degenerative brain disease affecting cognitive function in many areas of the brain. It's characterized by gradual memory loss, a decline in the ability to perform routine tasks, disorientation, learning difficulties, loss of language skills, impaired judgment, and personality changes.

As the number of cases of AD has grown, I've heard people in my office tell me that their understanding is that it's inevitable, that we're all going to get Alzheimer's eventually, right?

Wrong. While AD is a disease that occurs most frequently as we age—one in ten people aged sixty-five and older get the dementia associated with Alzheimer's disease—it is not an inevitable part of aging. We do know, however, that the older we get, the higher our risk grows. Specifically, at age sixty-five, the risk is one in twenty (5 percent), and by age eighty-five it is one in three (33 percent).

Some would argue that the rise of AD is a by-product of our advances in medicine in other areas that have enabled us to live longer and otherwise healthier lives. Some might even say that it's a price we pay for living longer.

That may be true, but if so, those affected are paying dearly.

Dr. Katzman used the right word in his 1976 paper describing the disease. The prevalence or incidence of Alzheimer's today is staggering. An estimated 5.5 million Americans were diagnosed with Alzheimer's dementia in 2017, according to the Alzheimer's Association, and approximately two hundred thousand people under age sixty-five are getting what's called early-onset Alzheimer's.[4]

It is also a disease to be feared, in large part because of its devastating course, which can start as benign forgetfulness, foretelling an insidious progression that ultimately ravages the mind as a whole and the body as well. The image of AD is searing and unforgettable, as Jamie can attest to. Her memory of seeing her great-grandmother has stuck with her for decades. Given the family's genetic structure, it is likely that she had Alzheimer's. But back then it was probably assumed that Grandma Neva was simply "senile" and that such a condition was simply a part of getting old.

We know better now. But what many people still confuse is the distinction between Alzheimer's and dementia. The two terms are often used interchangeably. Not so.

Dementia is the umbrella term for the loss of cognitive function, such as reasoning and memory, which is severe enough to interfere with daily life. Alzheimer's is a type of dementia, just as breast cancer is a type of a larger disease category, cancer.

And just as there are many forms of cancer, there are many types of dementia. The most prevalent is Alzheimer's, but there are others, including Lewy body dementia (comedian/actor Robin Williams is said to have had this), and frontotemporal dementia (also known as Pick's disease). Dementia can also be caused by a series of strokes, alcohol and drug abuse, or head trauma (a single injury or multiple blows), normal-pressure hydrocephalus (more commonly referred to as water on the brain), thyroid disorders, vitamin B12 deficiency, as well by AIDS and the lesser-known Creutzfeldt-Jakob disease (think mad cow for humans). People suffering from Parkinson's disease also often develop dementia.[5]

Just as dementia and Alzheimer's disease shouldn't be used interchangeably, I think it's important to recognize that Alzheimer's disease itself is a broad term. I think a lot of people believe that the disease is synonymous with the disturbing behaviors often associated with those in its later stages. But it's important to remember that Alzheimer's is a decades-long disease process that involves both biological changes (such as the formation of amyloid plaques) and clinical manifestations, the most recognizable being chronic forgetfulness.

Scientists are not absolutely sure why the changes that characterize AD begin, but they are sure that those plaques and tangles that Dr. Alois Alzheimer identified under the microscope over a century ago are a hallmark of the disease that bears his name.

What are these strange-sounding abnormalities? Plaques are abnormal clusters of chemically "sticky" proteins called beta-amyloid fragments that build up between nerve cells. In a healthy brain, these fragments are broken down and eliminated. In AD, amyloid plaques are insoluble clumps that accumulate in the brain and disrupt mental function. Tangles are made primarily of a protein called tau that accumulates within nerve cells in the brain, causing massive dysfunction and ultimately cell death.

While Dr. Alzheimer himself got the basics right, the changes to the brain in an Alzheimer's patient were not fully understood until the 1980s, when Dr. George Glenner and his colleagues at the University of California–San Diego and Dr. Wong established that the amyloid plaque or amyloid beta peptide was the core constituent cause of AD. This and other molecular, genetic, and pathological discoveries were advanced in the last two decades, which has improved our understanding of the disease and our research into treatments and, perhaps, even prevention.[6]

In a succession of discoveries, amyloid protein was found to come from a parent molecule known as an amyloid precursor protein. Not to get too deep in the biochemical weeds, but amyloid is a seminal catalyst, driving a cascade of events leading to dementia, including dysfunction of the synapses and increased plaque deposits, not to mention atrophy of key parts of the brain, such as the hippocampus and the cortex. Understanding why, in some individuals, amyloid is overproduced or under cleared—meaning that it is not removed at the normal expected rate—could be a critical step in our understanding of AD.

Another discovery involved identifying the fact that all people with Down's syndrome—a disorder arising from a chromosome defect, causing intellectual impairment and physical abnormalities—developed Alzheimer's disease in their lifetime, especially if they live past the age of forty. The next big breakthrough came in the ability of scientists to take genetically-engineered mice with mutations, which led them to develop Alzheimer's disease and amyloid a-beta production in the brain of the mice. A whole line of research has since focused on how the brain produces and processes amyloid, which are the main causes of toxic events and cell damage that eventually destroy the brain.

THE PROGRESSION OF AD

Earlier I talked about some of the optimism we in the research community are feeling about prevention and treatment of AD. Describing the progression of the disease, however, is a grim business. And perhaps it's not easy to read, especially if you're dealing with a loved one who may be showing signs of AD. But in order to determine the best treatment options, and, I would argue, in order to better fight back, it's still important to understand its workings and the course that AD typically takes. Below is a summary of the phases that Alzheimer's patients go through as they progress from mildly affected to advanced dementia.

Common Clinical Stages of Dementia Due to Alzheimer's Disease	
Mild Stage	
The symptoms commonly present in this stage are often mistaken for old age.	
Memory	*Poor recall of new information:* Experiences short-term memory loss, quickly forgetting new facts and occurrences and often repeating themselves. Long-term memory, or recall of things that happened in the distant past, is preserved. Simple, occasional forgetfulness is not a cause of alarm. As my colleague at Rush University, Dr. Robert Wilson, likes to say, and I'm paraphrasing: "The problem isn't when you forget where you put your house keys; it's when you forget where your house is."
Language	*Dysnomia (impaired naming of objects):* Has trouble recalling words and names, even familiar ones such as family members' names, to a far greater degree than those who experience normal age-related forgetfulness. *Mild loss of fluency:* Talks less over time.
Visuospatial	*Misplacing objects:* Frequently loses glasses, keys, and other objects. *Difficulty driving:* Has difficulty in perception and makes poor decisions while driving.

Behavioral	*Depression:* Frequently becoming depressed and withdrawn. Often early signs of Alzheimer's are mistaken for depression. But when the depression is treated, the cognitive impairment remains. *Anxiety:* People with Alzheimer's are often very anxious. This may be related to their short-term memory loss. Because of this, they tend to feel uncertain in situations that are not part of their regular routine.

Moderate Stage
Also referred to as moderate Alzheimer's. The symptoms of the moderate stage become apparent as AD progresses. This is often the stage when family members arrange care. People suffering from Alzheimer's are placed in long-term care for three principal reasons: behavioral problems, falling, and loss of bodily functions such as incontinence.

Memory	*Remote memory:* Confused with things happening in the past or present.
Language	*Nonfluent:* Loses the ability to produce language. *Poor comprehension:* Loses the ability to understand or follow conversations and instructions over time.
Visuospatial	*Getting lost:* May get lost, even in stores or places they have been many times before, including in their own neighborhood.
Behavioral	*Delusions:* Believes things have occurred when they have not. This is extremely distressing to family members. Examples include thinking something was stolen when it was simply lost. *Depression:* Loses interest in activities they once enjoyed. *Agitation:* Has verbal outbursts or physical threats for seemingly minor incidents or requests, such as bathing and eating. *Sleep:* Experiences sleep disturbances, which may be caused by the loss of the internal sleep regulation or the drive for sleep, excessive medication use, sleep-disordered breathing, depression, or chronic bed rest. Other sleep disturbances might include nocturnal wandering.

Neurological	*Reflexive grasping*: Grasps automatically, similar to infants, when something is placed in their palm and puckering of the lips in anticipation of being fed. Also known to neurologists as "snout reflex." *Parkinson's disease–like symptoms:* Stiff and slowed movement, and what we call "nonspecific gait disorder," which is walking slower than usual and walking that may require assistance.

Advanced Stage	
By this stage, many or most people with Alzheimer's are already in long-term care.	
Memory	*Severely impacted short-term and long-term memory:* May no longer recognize loved ones or remember large segments of their lives.
Language	*Lost language production:* They might lose the ability to talk to the point where their speech becomes largely unintelligible.
Behavioral	*Agitation:* Becomes easily agitated. This might include physical aggression toward caregivers as well as resistance toward basic activities such as bathing and dressing. *Wandering:* Tends to wander in the home, neighborhood, or to walk even great distances when unsupervised. *Loss of insight:* Denies having a disability. This can be distressing for families, especially when they try to point out a memory problem or an error in judgment.
Neurological	*Incontinence:* Loses control of bladder and bowel function. *Frontal release signs:* Reflexive grasping when something is place in the palm and puckering of the lips in anticipation of being fed. *Rigidity:* Becomes increasingly slow and stiff in movement. *Loss of gait:* Unable to walk and at the end of life cannot sit or hold themselves up.

Yes, it's a sad progress. And that slow but steady deterioration of the mind and body is why we call this a debilitating and progressive disease. But we're going to talk in future chapters about what you can do to alter or at least better manage this bleak forecast for you or your loved one.

CHAPTER 5

The Genetic Puzzle of AD

MARWAN SABBAGH, MD

I n the previous chapter, I mentioned some of those frequently asked questions I get from my patients or when I speak about Alzheimer's. Those adult children who have watched a parent suffer from the disease and are terrified by the possibility that they or their children will inherit it usually have two other questions that they're eager to ask:

1. Should I know my risk for Alzheimer's?
2. Do I *want* to know my risk for Alzheimer's?

It wasn't long ago that it would have been hard to assess this kind of risk. The science of genetics really exploded in 2003 with the release of the Human Genome Project, in which researchers mapped the 25,000 genes in the human genome.[1] This advance in genetic science produced a massive amount of collected data on DNA that is now benefiting many people. Genetic tests give us a glimpse into the DNA we inherited from our families: the good, the bad, and the terrifying. They're designed to look for hereditary genes hidden away in our DNA. Researchers can discover if there are any flaws in our genetic material that can cause a health condition. In some cases, these diseases can turn up immediately; in others they might manifest later in life.

When it comes to AD, the question of whether you should or would want to know your risk takes on new meaning to all of us after hearing Jamie's story. Let me tell you another one. A woman in her early thirties who came to see me with her husband seemed much too young to have a memory-impairment problem. She said, "You took care of my father when he had Alzheimer's. I'm married now, and we want to start a family. I want to know if I could pass it on to them."

I pulled out her father's chart and saw that, after he passed, his body went to the Brain and Body Donation Program at the Banner Sun Health Research Institute, where I was then research director—and where, as you have read, Jamie has participated in research. When I reviewed the autopsy report and the genetic analyses, I discovered that this young woman's father did *not* have any of the known genetic Alzheimer's mutations.

After I shared this good news, the woman and her husband started crying and thanking me, knowing that their future children's prospects were brighter. Her reaction is a reminder of the terror we have of this disease, not only for our parents or ourselves, but for our own kids.

Of course, not everyone gets such an encouraging genetic report as that woman. But the very fact that we have now added genetics to our diagnostic toolbox is a huge change, something that not only Dr. Alois Alzheimer but even some of the more recent pioneers in AD research couldn't have envisioned. Only in the last two decades have we been able to assess genetic risks for all kinds of diseases, and AD in particular. No longer is it just tangles and plaques that help us diagnose the disease or its stage; now we're looking at genes and chromosomes to help us predict, or at least assess the risk of getting AD in the first place.

Genetics, as you probably know, is one of the hottest fields in medicine. Scarcely a week goes by without some new study or discovery making the headlines that has emerged from our ever-evolving understanding of how inherited characteristics shape us as individuals.

So just as we reviewed the ABCs of Alzheimer's in the last chapter, perhaps a little Genetics 101 might be in order here.

Almost every human cell contains a "blueprint" that carries instructions, much like a job description. This blueprint is our DNA (or deoxyribonucleic acid), which contains proteins packed tightly together into compact structures called chromosomes. Each chromosome is broken into many thousands of segments, called genes.

We all inherit two copies of each gene from our parents (mom and dad genes, if you will). The one exception for genes is the X and Y chromosomes, which, among other functions, determine our gender. Genes are also involved in almost every aspect of a cell's construction, operation, and repair. Even slight changes in genes can increase or decrease the risk of developing a particular disease.

The genetic code behind a trait is known as the genotype. It refers to the entire set of genes in a cell, an organism, or an individual. A gene for a particular physical characteristic can exist in two alleles. An allele is one of a pair of genes that determines physical traits such as eye, skin, or hair color. When a dominant allele is paired with a recessive allele, the dominant one determines the characteristic.

Now here's where the myths and misconceptions of genetics can drive people (and their doctors) nuts. I've had patients in my office who are convinced they will get AD because one of their parents had it, and they happen to resemble that parent more than the other.

Regardless of whose appearance you may take after, the truth is that we are all a mixture of our mom and dad. Each parent contributes half of his or her own personal gene inventory to each child. One copy of each gene passes through the sperm, and one copy of each gene passes through the egg. So at each pregnancy, there is a 50 percent chance that the mutant gene will be passed along from the parent who has that gene. Physical resemblances such as eye color or skin type used to be taken as a sign that two people shared the same genes for other traits, including Alzheimer's. That's not the case, though, because all traits are inherited independently. Having red hair like your mom's doesn't mean you have also inherited her susceptibility for getting dementia.

Who you look like is not something I'm concerned about. For those of us who study and treat AD, a big red flag in the genes department is ApoE4 (or apolipoprotein E4). When this gene was discovered in 1993, researchers found that carriers had a higher lifetime risk for developing AD. As you've read, a double copy, which Jamie has (hence the "4/4" label), puts the lifetime risk of developing Alzheimer's at around 91 percent.

Now before we go labeling this gene as Public Enemy Number One, we should note that just as, say, fat can be both good and bad, the generic ApoE gene plays an important and beneficial role in human physiology.

Here, a little biochemistry is in order. The ApoE gene is part of a specific class of proteins called apolipoproteins. These have the specific task of capturing fats and other proteins out of the digestive track and transporting them to the liver. As such, ApoE helps to regulate our lipid, or fat, metabolism—overall, a good, healthy function.

We've mentioned the various subtypes of genes called alleles. In the case of the ApoE gene, these include Apo2, -3 and -4. You would get one gene from each parent, so you would be ApoE 2/2, 2/3, 3/3, and so on.

One of those subtypes, ApoE4, is a strong risk factor for developing AD. Thus, as one researcher concluded, "It is reasonable to assume that lipids such as cholesterol are involved" in the development of AD. In fact, up to 60 percent of all people with late-onset Alzheimer's are ApoE4 carriers. People who develop Alzheimer's are more likely to have an ApoE4 allele than people who do not develop the disease. Dozens of studies have confirmed that the presence of the ApoE4 allele increases the risk of developing age-related cognitive decline and Alzheimer's disease but, again, scientists still do not understand why this happens. We do know, however, that when ApoE4 lipoproteins bind to cell-surface receptors to deliver lipids, it causes connections between brain cells to break down, the same kind of degeneration we see in cases of AD.

It's also worth noting that variants of ApoE have been studied extensively as potential risk factors for different conditions, including cardiovascular diseases. People who carry at least one copy of the ApoE4 allele have an increased chance of developing atherosclerosis, an accumulation of fatty deposits and scarlike tissue in the lining of the arteries. This progressive narrowing of the arteries can lead to a heart attack or stroke.

As complex as all of this may sound, it's also part of what's fascinating about genetics and its critical role for researchers like me trying to get to the bottom of AD. ApoE is necessary for good health. But add a "4" and it's a potential health risk. Double it to two ApoE4 genes and you're talking a 91 percent risk of AD.

Here is the silver lining, though, for Jamie and everyone else who has this gene or two of them. Not all people with Alzheimer's disease have the ApoE4 allele, and not all people who have this allele will develop the disease. Some people with one or two ApoE4 alleles never get the disease, and others who develop Alzheimer's do not have any ApoE4 alleles. In other words, there are no absolutes here.

So that brings us back to the question: Do I need to get tested for my risk of AD? We are going to discuss the pros and cons of this complicated decision in the next chapter. But let me leave you here with words of hope, words like those I offered to Jamie when we met.

If you or a family member is at risk or have been diagnosed with the disease, our goal here is to help you understand the big picture ahead and encourage you to begin the necessary planning. Though it may sometimes seem that this is a path strewn with nothing but despair, keep in mind this famous quote by Desmond Tutu, the South African cleric and Nobel Peace Prize winner: "Hope is being able to see that there is light despite all of the darkness." It is only a matter of time before the research community finds a prevention and/or treatment for this terrible disease. Thanks in large part to what we're learning from genetics, I believe that time is coming sooner rather than later.

There is certainly light to be found in the impressive new interventions and drugs that I'll detail later in this book, all of which are poised to help us begin a new paradigm in the treatment of AD. In the meantime, as I said to Jamie that day I met her, keep the faith! She certainly has, even under trying circumstances, and I'm sure you will too.

CHAPTER 6

To Test or Not to Test

MARWAN SABBAGH, MD

While genetic testing may sound complex, the procedure is actually quite simple. DNA is collected from saliva, blood, or a cheek swab. A lab then analyzes the number, arrangement, and characteristics of the chromosomes in the DNA and identifies abnormal and mutated genes as well as markers for inherited diseases, including Alzheimer's.[1]

The results of these tests can be used to help diagnose diseases such as AD, identify gene mutations that are the cause of a diagnosed disease, determine the severity of a disease, identify gene changes that may increase the risk and probability of developing the disease, and they may help allow physicians to prescribe the best medicine or treatment available. These tests can also identify gene changes that could be passed on to children, screen newborn babies for certain treatable conditions, and trace ancestry.

Clearly, these exciting, useful tools have opened up a new frontier for medicine. But these tests can also be problematic, as Jamie's experience reminds us. The reason she signed up to take a genetic test was to deter-mine whether or not she had MS, which was one of the diseases being tested for in the study she agreed to participate in. She found instead that she had two sets of the ApoE4 gene we discussed in the last chapter, which suggests an extremely high probability that she could develop AD.

Of course, it's not inevitable, and there are other factors that could affect her future. But she didn't know that, sitting in her home office, reading the results on a printout. All she saw was that she had a 91 per-cent chance of getting Alzheimer's. That's not how anyone should get this information, especially someone with a family history of AD!

Let's say you had breast cancer running in your family. No oncolo-gist would do a BRCA test (to identify the breast cancer gene) without advising you to have genetic counseling or explaining the importance of the test. The doctor's office might even schedule a meeting with the counselor. The same thing should have happened with Jamie.

WHAT DO DOCTORS LOOK FOR IN GENETIC TESTS?

Inheriting a disease, condition, or trait depends on the type of chromo-some affected as well as whether the trait is dominant or recessive. One thing physicians look for is a genetic predisposition (sometimes called genetic susceptibility), which is an increased likelihood of developing a particular disease based on your genetic makeup. A genetic predisposi-tion results from specific gene variations that are often inherited from a parent. This includes what's called "autosomal dominant disease," which is one of several ways that a trait or disorder can be passed down, or inherited, in families. An example of an autosomal dominant disease includes Huntington's disease (HD), a condition in which nerve cells in certain parts of the brain waste away or degenerate.[2] In an autosomal dominant disease like HD, if you inherit a single dominant abnormal gene from only one parent, you have a 100 percent chance of getting the disease.[3] Often, one of the parents may also have the disease. In other words, if you have an autosomal dominant gene, there is a virtual certainty you will get that disease, and if you don't have that gene, there is a virtual certainty you won't get that disease.

ApoE4 is not an autosomal dominant gene, so there are no absolutes when it comes to AD risk, but in either case, getting a genetic counselor, should you decide to get tested, is highly recommended. Had I known Jamie at the time, I would have advised her not to participate in the study if the results were not accompanied by genetic counseling.

Additionally, genes are inherited, so a first-degree relative (mother, father, sister, brother) can double or even triple the person's risk of developing AD—although, I hasten to add, not in every case.[4]

SHOULD YOU TAKE THE TEST?

When a genetic test reveals information about an individual, there is a likelihood that others in the family might also have that same gene. In other words, a genetic test of one person can actually be a test of an entire family. Given that someone who has received disturbing news about his or her status might feel obligated to tell family members, this can literally create bad blood among relatives who might blame the person who passed along the flawed gene. Because all ApoE4 genotypes are inherited, before you start looking up your family tree, understand that you might be a carrier.

In any event, I believe that if someone has symptoms of memory loss and cognitive decline, it should be up to the patient and his or her doctor to decide whether to get tested. Whatever you decide to do, talking to a geneticist or genetic counselor beforehand can help you weigh the pros and cons of testing for AD. Genetic counselors will talk with individuals and families about the scientific, emotional, and ethical factors associated with the decision to have genetic testing and how best to deal with the results of the test should you decide to have one.

IS IGNORANCE BLISS?

In my previous chapter I told you that one of the most common questions I get from patients is, "Should I even *want* to learn my genetic status?" There are some who decide they don't want to know. That's certainly understandable. But consider this: a recent study from the University of California–Los Angeles showed that approximately forty-seven million Americans are walking around with no symptoms but have AD brain pathology or are presymptomatic, stage 1 AD. Having an ApoE4 status can help doctors to determine the probability of your developing AD if you or a loved one is exhibiting what we call "clinical symptoms of mild cognitive impairment or predementia," meaning your memory loss is noticeable but not so severe that it affects your daily life (which would be the case for someone with dementia).

Knowing your genetic status might be a great motivator to make some of the lifestyle modifications that we know can help delay the development of AD. It might also encourage you to start enjoying life to its fullest rather than letting the little problems get in the way or to make the appropriate plans for the future, such as getting long-term care insurance before testing.

There are some other things you might want to keep in mind, as well, as you consider genetic testing. First, if you have mild cognitive impairment and you are an ApoE4 carrier, the probability of progressing to dementia is three times greater per year than if you don't carry the ApoE4 gene. Second, and the most worrisome, is if you are an ApoE4 carrier with symptoms of progressive dementia, the probability of your having the pathological features of Alzheimer's—the plaques and tangles and shrinkage in certain parts of the brain—increases to 97 percent. As a doctor, knowing the probabilities makes me more confident about diagnosis, which allows me to treat accordingly.[5]

TO KNOW OR NOT TO KNOW: CONFLICTING STUDIES ON THE IMPACT

In a 2009 *New England Journal of Medicine* article, researchers involved with the Risk Evaluation and Education for Alzheimer's (REVEAL) study published a paper showing, essentially, that adult children of Alzheimer's patients were able to shrug off the presence of the ApoE gene in their own makeup. "The disclosure of *ApoE* genotyping results to adult children of patients with Alzheimer's disease did not result in significant short-term psychological risks," the 2009 study concluded. "Test-related distress was reduced among those who learned that they were ApoE-negative. Persons with high levels of emotional distress before undergoing genetic testing were more likely to have emotional difficulties after disclosure."[6]

In contrast, another study that appeared in a 2014 issue of *The American Journal of Psychology* found that telling people they are carriers did have an adverse impact on their emotional well-being.[7] The conflicting results of these two studies suggest the complexities involved. That reinforces my belief that genetic testing is a personal decision based on the circumstances of your life, your health, and your family. It's a decision that you, your family, your doctor, and your genetic counselor must discuss before taking that medical leap. In any case, having genetic counseling prior to testing can help reduce your anxiety concerning their ApoE4 status.

WHY CONSIDER GENETIC TESTING?

While I'm not trying to persuade you to get tested, and I certainly understand those who opt out, I would like to point out some reasons why I often recommend it to my patients.

For some, genetic testing can be a wake-up call. Knowing one's status might be just the spark you need to finally quit smoking, to start getting physically active, to modify your diet and lose a few pounds—things that are good for your health in general and that have also been shown to help decrease or delay the risk of AD.

Remember also that it often takes twenty years of changes in the brain before people with Alzheimer's exhibit symptoms of dementia. This means that by the time a person demonstrates those clinical symptoms, changes in the brain have been going on for a while. If you're at risk, the need to make lifestyle changes as soon as possible is imperative. If genetic testing is the prod that will get you to do that, I'm all for it.

There is a caveat here when it comes to AD: while I routinely and vigorously encourage my patients to adopt a healthier lifestyle, I separate prevention from treatment. Changes in lifestyle can help people at risk, but, sadly, lifestyle changes are less likely to improve the condition of people already experiencing cognitive impairment or dementia.

Knowing your status could also give you the opportunity to enlist in clinical trials to find a treatment or cure for people with the ApoE4 gene. There are genetic tests and clinical trials for numerous diseases, some well-known, some rare. Let me share one of the most inspiring examples of how a family decided to use the results of a genetic test to help others, knowing full well it probably wouldn't be able to help them. This particular story has nothing to do with Alzheimer's but everything to do with the spirit of helping others and contributing to the greater good.

In January 2018, Richard Engel, chief foreign correspondent for NBC News, related on the *Today* show the heartrending story of genetic testing and his young son Henry. Engel was on assignment with US troops in South Korea when he received results of a full set of genetic tests for his son. In what he calls "the worst day of his life," Engel and his wife learned that Henry had a rare genetic brain disorder called Rett syndrome. There is currently no treatment or cure for Rett. The couple knew early on that something wasn't right with their son when, at age two, Henry couldn't talk, walk, sit up straight, or clap his hands. Doctors told the parents that their son would probably never be able to dress himself and that his mental capacity would likely remain at the toddler level. The couple was also warned about future health problems, such as seizures and rigidity.[8]

Here's the good news for this sweet, adorable child and his devoted parents: Henry's unique mutation is now being studied with the hope of finding the key to a treatment for him and others. The work is being conducted by Dr. Huda Zoghbi, director of the Duncan Neurological Research Institute at Texas Children's Hospital in Houston, the same researcher who helped discover the mutation that causes Rett syndrome.[9] As Dr. Zoghbi told the *Today* show, "We now know there are hundreds of genes that can cause autism or can cause intellectual disability or complex psychiatric disorders. Using Henry's cells to study Rett syndrome, when successful, can be applied to any of those diseases."

Engel had the courage to share this on national television. "It's not a story that anybody wants to tell," he said. "It is very difficult for us, but we wanted to raise awareness, to make other families with special needs children, children who are challenging, know that they're not alone."[10]

Similarly, I know of many families and patients with Alzheimer's who have taken the knowledge they learned from genetic tests, through participation in clinical trials and other forms of research, and used it to help others. One such person, of course, is Jamie, whose exemplary decision to volunteer as a research participant once she learned of her 4/4 genetic status made a difference for others.

Jamie and others who do the same know full well they will probably not be the ones helped by whatever is learned from the studies they are participating in. The beneficiaries of the medical knowledge gleaned through that research will be others, made possible by their selfless behavior. At a time when finding subjects is one of the biggest challenges for those of us who do research in Alzheimer's, we're grateful to people like Jamie and others who volunteer to participate. If you or a member of your family are genetically tested and find you are a carrier of the ApoE4 gene, I certainly hope you will consider following their lead. (More information on how to find genetic counseling can be found on the website of the National Society of Genetic Counselors, www.nsgc.org.)

HOW MUCH DO GENETIC TESTS COST?

The average genetic testing costs range from ninety-nine dollars for commercial testing to north of two thousand, when looking for a rare mutation like Rett. Depending on the reason for the test, your health insurance carrier might not cover all or even part of the cost.

Most people are not aware that testing for the ApoE is actually a cardiology test, which is what it was originally used for. This is significant, because it is cheaper to do a cardiac test for the ApoE4 gene ($99) than it is to do an Alzheimer's test at $399. It's all a matter of how the healthcare provider codes when billing. It should also be noted that some people inadvertently discover their risk for AD because their cardiologist tested for cardiac risk, a complete surprise to the patient, who leaves the office filled with anxiety. Discuss this with your physician if you are thinking of getting tested for ApoE4.

And if you are thinking of getting tested, I recommend you do it through your physician or a lab he or she refers you to. While there is much interesting, fun, and often useful information to be learned from the home genetic tests that are now popular, the lack of genetic counseling it provides is not ideal, and Jamie's experience should serve as a sobering reminder of the perils of this method when it comes to assessing your risk of AD.

PROBLEMS OF HOME GENETIC TESTING

The following is a cautionary tale about how reports are coming out that consumer genetic tests are far from foolproof and may be scaring their users with false results. On a lark, Julie Kennerly-Shah, a pharmacist, and Dr. Summit Shah told a reporter from the *Huffington Post* that they decided to buy kits from 23andMe for fun in 2016 while they were dating. The Ohio-based couple wanted to learn more about their heritage, and they were curious to see what it had to say about their health.[11]

After sending their data to Promethease, a third-party DNA analysis company that examines people's DNA to map out a genetic family tree, they were unfazed by the results. In January 2018, however, when the then-newlyweds logged back onto Promethease, they were shocked to discover that Kennerley-Shah had a gene mutation linked to Lynch syndrome, a rare genetic condition that gives people a more than 80 percent risk of developing colon cancer and gives women a 71 percent risk of endometrial cancer. The report also detected a genetic heart disease that increases her risk of arrhythmias and sudden death, even in people with no symptoms. As a doctor at Ohio State University's Comprehensive Cancer Center, Kennerly-Shah was familiar with this devastating genetic condition, but she said her husband was "probably more scared than I was, and I think that probably increased my anxiety." The couple's future in flux, they decided to try to get pregnant sooner than they had planned, as hysterectomies are often recommended as preventive measures for women with Lynch syndrome, and considered IVF so they could monitor the genes of the implanted embryos.

Fortunately, this story has a happy ending. On the advice of colleagues,

Kennerly-Shah scheduled an appointment with a genetic counselor at the Ohio State University Wexner Medical Center to confirm her genetic status. The hospital's results came back negative, meaning she did not have the genetic mutations for Lynch syndrome and that Promethease had given them a false positive report. Unfortunately, this story is not unusual. A study by Ambry Genetics, a clinical diagnostics company, found that 40 percent of forty-nine direct-to-consumer reports reanalyzed using clinical-grade lab testing were actually false positives.

The only direct-to-consumer genetic test authorized by the FDA to provide reports on genetic risk is 23andMe, which has more than two million customers. The founders of the lesser-used Promethease told the *Huffington Post* it gives out five hundred reports a day, but neither company would share its data on how many results are false positives. The likely prospect of getting incorrect information about your health raises further questions about the validity of DIY genetic tests.[12]

After examining home genetic tests currently on the market, *Consumer Reports* concluded: "The most accurate way to get information about your genetic health risks is still through tests that a doctor (often an oncologist or OB-GYN) orders for you. These tests tend to be far more comprehensive than those that can be purchased over the counter because they usually sequence entire genes and look for many variants that have been linked to the disease in question."[13]

Genetic testing done at home is becoming more and more commonplace. We have summarized here the pitfalls and perils of home testing and the fact that in many cases physicians and patients aren't well equipped to deal with the complexity and gravity of the data that's handed to them. So I think if you want to know who your relatives might be based on DNA or want to find out the name of your great-grandmother five times removed, enjoy the rich bounty of information these websites provide. But if you really want to know your risk for AD, it's best done in collaborative fashion with your neurologist.

CHAPTER 7

Don't Forget the Other Tests

MARWAN SABBAGH, MD

The previous chapter was all about genetic testing. But of course, genetic tests are not the only ways to assess whether someone has Alzheimer's. Very often, we're looking for other biomarkers. The National Institute on Aging, an excellent resource for information, offers a glossary of the various types of biomarkers and tests. While you've probably heard of some of them, this might give you a better understanding of the whys and wherefores. I've included some observations based on my own research and experience as well.

First, just to make sure we're clear on our terms, biomarkers are a measure of what is happening inside the living body, shown by the results of laboratory and imaging tests. Biomarkers can help doctors and scientists diagnose diseases and health conditions, find health risks in a person, monitor responses to treatment, and see how a person's disease or health condition changes over time. For example, an increased level of cholesterol in the blood is interpreted as a biomarker for heart-attack risk.

Many types of biomarker tests are used for research on Alzheimer's disease and related dementias. Changes in the brains of people with these disorders may begin many years before memory loss or other symptoms appear. Researchers use biomarkers to help detect these brain changes in people, who may or may not yet have obvious changes in memory or thinking. Finding these changes early in the disease process helps identify people who are at the greatest risk of Alzheimer's or another dementia and may help determine which people might benefit most from a particular treatment.

TYPES OF BIOMARKERS AND TESTS

In Alzheimer's disease and related dementias, the most widely used biomarkers measure changes in the size and function of the brain and its parts, as well as levels of certain proteins seen on brain scans and in cerebrospinal fluid and blood.

Brain Imaging

Brain imaging, also called brain scans, can measure changes in the size of the brain, identify and measure specific brain regions, and detect biochemical changes and vascular damage (damage related to blood vessels). In clinical settings, doctors can use brain scans to find evidence of brain disorders, such as tumors or strokes that may aid in diagnosis. In research settings, brain imaging is used to study structural and biochemical changes in the brain in Alzheimer's disease and related dementias. There are several types of brain scans.

Computerized Tomography

A computerized tomography (CT) scan is a type of X-ray that uses radiation to produce images of the brain. During a CT, a person lies in a scanner for five to ten minutes. A doughnut-shaped device moves around the head to produce the image.

A CT can show the size of the brain and identify a tumor, stroke, head injury, or other potential cause of dementia symptoms. CT scans provide greater detail than traditional X-rays, but a less detailed picture than magnetic resonance imaging (MRI) and cannot easily measure changes over time. Sometimes a CT scan is used when people can't get an MRI due to metal in their body, such as a pacemaker. A CT is typically used in dementia and Alzheimer's to exclude the possibility of a tumor, stroke, or water on the brain.

Magnetic Resonance Imaging

Magnetic resonance imaging (MRI) uses magnetic fields to produce detailed images of body structures, including the size and shape of the brain and brain regions. Doctors often use MRI scans to identify or rule out causes of memory loss, such as a stroke or other vascular brain injury, tumors, or hydrocephalus. These scans also can be used to assess shrinkage of specific regions of the brain.

During an MRI, a person lies still in a tunnel-shaped scanner for about thirty to forty-five minutes for diagnostic purposes and up to two hours for research purposes. MRI is a safe, painless procedure that does not involve radioactivity. The procedure is noisy, so people are often given earplugs or headphones to wear. Some people become claustrophobic and anxious inside an MRI machine, which can be addressed with anxiety-relieving medication taken shortly before the scan. Because MRI uses strong magnetic fields to obtain images, people with certain types of metal in their bodies, such as a pacemaker, surgical clips, or shrapnel, cannot undergo the procedure.

An MRI scan provides clearer pictures of brain structures than a CT and can help tell us whether abnormal changes, such as shrinkage (or atrophy) of areas of the brain, are present. Evidence of shrinkage in certain areas may support a diagnosis of Alzheimer's or another neurode-generative dementia but cannot indicate a specific diagnosis. Researchers use different types of MRI scans to obtain pictures of brain structure, chemistry, blood flow, and function, as well as the size of brain regions. MRI also provides a detailed picture of any vascular damage in the brain, such as damage due to a stroke or small areas of bleeding that may contribute to changes in cognition. Repeat scans can show how a person's brain changes over time.

In the research arena, various types of MRI scans are used to study the structure and function of the brain in aging and Alzheimer's disease. In clinical trials, MRI can be used to monitor the safety of novel drugs and to examine how treatment may affect the brain structure and volume over time.

PET Scans

Positron emission tomography (PET) uses small amounts of a radioactive substance, called a tracer, to measure specific activity—such as glucose (energy) use—in different brain regions. Different PET scans use different tracers. PET is commonly used in dementia research. In clinical settings, it is generally used for cancer staging and to detect if a cancer is spreading.

The person having a PET scan of the brain receives an injection of a radioactive tracer into a vein in the arm, then lies on a cushioned table, which is moved into a doughnut-shaped scanner. The PET scanner takes pictures of the brain, revealing regions of normal and abnormal chemical activity. A PET scan is much quieter than an MRI. The entire process, including the injection and scan, takes about one hour. Patients can only have three PET scans a year because of radiation. Those who are concerned about radiation exposure or who have had many X-rays or imaging scans should talk with their doctor.

There are several specific types of PET scans used in the testing for Alzheimer's disease and dementias:

- Fluorodeoxyglucose (FDG) PET scans measure glucose use in the brain. Glucose, a type of sugar, is the primary source of energy for cells. Studies show that people with dementia often have abnormal patterns of decreased glucose use in specific areas of the brain. An FDG PET scan can show a pattern that may support a diagnosis of a specific cause of dementia.
- Amyloid PET scans measure abnormal deposits of a protein called beta-amyloid. Higher levels of beta-amyloid are consistent with the presence of amyloid plaques, a hallmark of Alzheimer's disease. Several tracers may be used for amyloid PET scans, including florbetapir, flutemetamol, florbetaben, and Pittsburgh compound B.
- Tau PET scans detect abnormal accumulation of the protein tau, which forms tangles in nerve cells of those with Alzheimer's disease or many other dementias. Several tau tracers are currently being studied in clinical trials and other research settings.

In clinical care, FDG PET scans may be used if a doctor strongly suspects frontotemporal dementia as opposed to Alzheimer's dementia based on the person's symptoms or when there is an unusual presentation of symptoms.

Amyloid PET imaging is sometimes used by medical specialists to help with a diagnosis when Alzheimer's disease is suspected but uncertain, even after a thorough evaluation. Amyloid PET imaging may also help with a diagnosis when people with dementia have unusual or very mild symptoms, an early age of onset (under age sixty-five), or any of several different conditions, such as severe depression, which may contribute to dementia symptoms. A negative amyloid PET scan rules out Alzheimer's disease.

In research, amyloid and tau PET scans are used to determine which individuals may be at greatest risk for developing Alzheimer's disease, to determine eligibility of participation for clinical trials, and to assess the impact of experimental drugs designed to affect amyloid or tau pathways.

Cerebrospinal Fluid Biomarkers

Cerebrospinal fluid (CSF) is a clear fluid that surrounds the brain and spinal cord, providing protection and insulation. CSF also supplies numerous nutrients and chemicals that help keep brain cells healthy. Proteins and other substances made by cells can be detected in CSF, and their levels may change years before symptoms of Alzheimer's and other brain disorders appear.

CSF is obtained by a lumbar puncture, also called a spinal tap, an outpatient procedure used to diagnose several types of neurological problems.

The phrase *spinal tap* makes some people cringe, but there's nothing to be afraid of. The modern spinal tap, if done properly, is a very safe, quick, and relatively painless office procedure.

During a lumbar puncture, the patient either sits or lies curled up on her side while the skin over the lower part of the spine is cleaned and injected with a local anesthetic. A thin needle is then inserted into the space between the bones of the lumbar region of the spine. CSF either drips out through the needle or is gently drawn out through a syringe. The procedure typically takes five to ten minutes. Some people feel brief pain during the procedure, but most have little discomfort.

After the procedure, the patient lies down for a few minutes and may receive something to eat or drink. People can drive themselves home and resume regular activities, but they should refrain from strenuous exercise for about twenty-four hours. A few may have a mild headache afterward, which usually disappears after taking a pain reliever and lying down. Sometimes, people develop a persistent headache that gets worse when they sit or stand. It's important to contact your doctor if you experience this, because this type of headache can be easily treated with a blood patch, which involves injecting a small amount of the person's blood into his or her lower back to stop a leak of CSF.

Certain people cannot have a lumbar puncture, including people who take medication such as warfarin (Coumadin or Jantoven) to thin their blood, have a low platelet count or an infection in the lower back, or have had major back surgery.

The most widely used CSF biomarkers for Alzheimer's disease measure certain proteins: beta-amyloid 42 (the major component of amyloid plaques in the brain), tau, and phospho-tau (major components of tau tangles in the brain). In Alzheimer's disease, beta-amyloid 42 levels in CSF are low, and tau and phospho-tau levels are high, compared with levels in people without Alzheimer's or other causes of dementia. Other markers—new proteins—are being developed that can show the difference between those with AD and without.

In clinical practice, CSF biomarkers may be used to help diagnose Alzheimer's, for example, in cases involving an unusual presentation of symptoms or course of progression. CSF also can be used to evaluate people with unusual types of dementia or with rapidly progressive dementia. In research, CSF biomarkers are valuable tools for early detection of a neurodegenerative disease. They are also used in clinical trials to assess the impact of experimental medications.

Blood Tests

Proteins that originate in the brain, such as tau and beta-amyloid 42, might be measured with sensitive blood tests. Levels of these proteins may change as a result of Alzheimer's, a stroke, or other brain disorders. These blood biomarkers are less well developed than CSF biomarkers for identifying Alzheimer's and related dementias. However, new methods to measure these brain-derived proteins, particularly beta-amyloid 42 and tau, have improved, suggesting that blood tests may be used in the future for screening and perhaps diagnosis.

Many other proteins, lipids, and other substances can be measured in the blood, but so far none has shown value in diagnosing Alzheimer's. Currently, dementia researchers use blood biomarkers to study early detection, prevention, and the effects of potential treatments. They are not yet available for use in doctors' offices and other clinical settings.

I'd like to emphasize two important points about testing overall. First, it's highly individualized. Second, it's very precise. Yes, some believe that we can only diagnose AD with an autopsy. Not true. Our precision in diagnosis is now extraordinarily high. We're not guessing anymore. As we've just discussed, a physician today has many tools at his or her disposal to help make a diagnosis. A good practitioner will use the tests that are right for the patient.

CHAPTER 8

The Real Risks of Alzheimer's

MARWAN SABBAGH, MD

O ur bodies are like engines; when we put lots of mileage on them, things can break down, especially if we don't give them the right fuel and proper maintenance. The science surrounding the risks and causes of Alzheimer's disease is robust and ongoing. And while I would like to ultimately put myself out of business by finding a cure, as yet, this cure has eluded us.

We do know, however, that multiple factors contribute to the development of the disease. Some are *modifiable*, risks that can be reduced or eliminated through lifestyle, dietary changes, or medication. Others are *unmodifiable*, such as your age or genetic structure.

While there is no real cure or prevention for AD, there are current treatments and lifestyle recommendations that have been shown to be effective in slowing down the progression of the disease or in decreasing your risk of getting it.

Earlier, we looked closely at genetic risks. But here are some of the others.

Let's start with some of the most common risk factors for Alzheimer's disease that cannot be modified.

Age

There has been much discussion about the genetic risks of AD. But let's not forget the most basic one: age. Advanced age is the strongest risk factor for Alzheimer's; the older you live, the higher your risk. By age sixty-five, 5 percent of people have AD. This risk doubles every five years. By age eighty-five, the risk of getting AD has been quoted as being as high as 50 percent. Personally, I think 33 percent is a more accurate number, which goes up to a 40 percent risk of AD at age ninety.

But, again, it is quite possible to reach a ripe old age without ever experiencing symptoms of AD. At my former research institute in Sun City, Arizona, we saw participants who ranged in age from their eighties to a hundred whose memories were as sharp as millennials'. By studying the healthy brains of the elderly, we hope to find the secret to maintaining normal cognition throughout our lifetime.

One reason for the increased risk of AD as we age is caused by what we call neuronal energy failure. All cells need energy to maintain healthy function, and the brain requires a great deal of energy. As we age, our brain cells become less efficient. To counteract this brain power outage, scientists are working to develop drugs that could enhance the function of the mitochondria cellular organelles (specialized structures within a cell that are rich in fats, proteins, and enzymes). But it's important to note that, so far, none of these mitochondrial drugs have proven effective.

Gender

It is perhaps also sadly fitting that the first patient identified as having what would be known as Alzheimer's disease was a woman, Auguste Deter, whose brain plaques and tangles were seen by Dr. Alois Alzheimer under his microscope in the early 1900s.

We know now that women have a greater risk than men of getting AD by a 60:40 ratio. Why? One reason is that women tend to live longer than men—although, interestingly enough, that ratio still exists even after adjusting for age. Another possible cause is that estrogen may be lost in the brains of women with AD. Because men use testosterone to make low levels of estrogen their entire lives, this doesn't seem to be a problem for them, but for women, the loss of estrogen over time could be a contributing cause of AD.

In a study conducted by Banner Sun Health Research Institute and the University of Chicago, the brains of women who died with AD showed much less estrogen content than those of the same age in the control group. Likewise, animal studies found that estrogen deficiency accelerates amyloid production and cognitive decline.

One might think that estrogen-infused hormone replacement therapy (HRT) might protect women from developing Alzheimer's, but large-scale studies have shown the opposite to be true. For example, the Women's Health Initiative showed that HRT is good for treatment of symptoms of menopause and for bone health related to osteoporosis. However, it still continued to show slight increased risks for certain types of cancer and potential cardiovascular risk and showed no protection against AD.

Ethnicity

For reasons that are not fully understood, Latinos are 50 percent more likely to be affected by AD than non-Latino whites. African Americans also have higher rates of AD.

MODIFIABLE RISKS

The good thing about modifiable risks is that, well, they can be modified! In other words, genes don't tell the whole story; environmental factors and lifestyle also play a role. The great news is that there is something you can do about these modifiable risks that can help slow down or possibly prevent certain AD risk factors.

Diabetes and Alzheimer's

What does diabetes have to do with Alzheimer's? Plenty. Type 2 diabetes (T2D), the most common form of diabetes, is associated with obesity, old age, family history, and inactivity. It is a condition in which the cells themselves resist the entry of blood sugar, even when there is adequate insulin in the blood. This insulin resistance is a key component of T2D, and it is the primary culprit when it comes to the risk of dementia and Alzheimer's. Both types increase glucose levels, and, if left untreated, can also cause severe damage to internal organs, particularly the kidneys, the eyes (especially the retinas), and the nerves. In a condition called diabetic peripheral neuropathy, the nerves in the feet are damaged, causing a lack of balance or a persistent burning sensation.[1]

The body of data we have about diabetes is good and growing, and this much is clear: T2D has strong links to both the onset of dementia, cognitive decline, and the risk of developing AD in both middle and old age. In fact, someone diagnosed with diabetes has about twice the risk of developing AD as does a nondiabetic. If you are a woman and/or have the ApoE4 gene, then your risk is even higher.

Why the connection between T2D and AD? Think about it this way: Our brains need a near-constant supply of glucose (blood sugar) in order to function, and insulin is a key player in providing and regulating this supply to the brain. Insulin is also responsible for regulating the activity in the brain cells themselves, as well as communicating signals from one neuron to another. Insulin is constantly transported across the blood/brain barrier (a semipermeable membrane that separates the blood from the brain and fluid in the central nervous system). When insulin and glucose metabolism are impaired, there is cognitive function and memory loss, and an increased risk of Alzheimer's disease, especially in people with type 2 diabetes.

In a 2015 University of California–San Francisco and Kaiser Permanente study, those with T2D were 50 to 100 percent more likely to develop dementia than those without T2D. Another study from the Kaiser Permanente Group of Northern California found a connection between high levels of glycosylated hemoglobin and a risk of developing Alzheimer's. Hemoglobin is the substance inside red blood cells that carries oxygen to the cells of the body. When glucose in the blood becomes stuck to hemoglobin, the hemoglobin becomes *glycosylated*, also referred to as HbA1c. Patients with a high HbA1c (greater than 15 percent) had a 78 percent greater risk of developing AD or cognitive decline within ten years. Patients with mild elevations of HbA1c had a 16 to 25 percent elevated risk. If you are diabetic, it's important to talk to your doctor about monitoring your HbA1c levels.[2]

While scientists are still not clear about what causes diabetes, we do know that the type 2 epidemic in America is likely the result of eating too much of the wrong types of foods (processed and high in sugar) combined with the lack of exercise. Here are some things you can do about that, and in turn, you may be helping to avoid or delay AD in the future.

- *Monitor.* Because of the numerous problems and health risks that come with type 2, it is important to have your glucose, cholesterol, blood pressure, and HbA1c regularly checked by your doctor. If you have diabetes, manage it meticulously. Your target blood sugar should be 70 to 110, and your target HbA1c should be less than 6.6.

- **Medicate.** You can also manage your diabetes with medication, if your doctor prescribes one for you. Metformin (Glucophage, Glumetza, and others) is generally the first medication prescribed for T2D. It works by improving the sensitivity of your tissues to insulin so that your body uses insulin more effectively. Metformin also lowers glucose production in the liver.

Like metformin, thiazolidinediones—which include rosiglitazone (Avandia) and pioglitazone (Actos)—make the body's tissues more sensitive to insulin. However, this class of medications has also been linked to weight gain and other more serious side effects, such as an increased risk of heart failure and fractures. Because of these risks, these are generally not a first-choice treatment.[3]

It's worth noting here that both of these medications have been researched as possible treatments for AD.

Of course there are other ways to treat and monitor your diabetes that don't involve medication: lifestyle! We'll talk more about that in upcoming chapters.

Alzheimer's As "Type 3" Diabetes

Researcher Suzanne de la Monte, MD, a professor of pathology, neurology, and neurosurgery at Rhode Island Hospital and the Alpert Medical School at Brown University, was one of the first to discover the association between a high-fat diet and insulin resistance in brain cells. She found that when she disrupted the way rats' brains respond to insulin, they developed the same kind of brain damage seen in Alzheimer's disease, with areas of the brain associated with memory clogged up with amyloid plaques. The plaques severed the connections between neurons, leaving brain cells on the verge of death. The rats were unable to learn how to navigate their way through a maze and stumbled around aimlessly.

In 2008, following this discovery, de la Monte published a paper in the *Journal of Diabetes Science and Technology*, stating that Alzheimer's is another form of diabetes, which she characterized as "type 3." She and her colleague concluded that the term type 3 diabetes accurately reflects the fact that AD is a form of diabetes that selectively involves the brain and has molecular and biochemical features that overlap with both type 1 and type 2. This theory could help explain why people with type 2 diabetes—a disease that plagues more than twenty-five million Americans—are significantly more likely to develop Alzheimer's. Given the link between AD and diabetes mellitus (DM), this suggests that targeting metabolism might be a way forward in the future.

Body Weight and Obesity

There is solid evidence that obesity, or a body mass index (BMI) of thirty or higher, might play a significant role in cognitive decline and dementia, including the development of Alzheimer's disease. This link has been demonstrated particularly when obesity first appears in middle age. Obesity also increases your risk for other conditions and diseases, including high blood pressure (hypertension), type 2 diabetes, heart disease, and arthritis. Like diabetes, obesity is a national epidemic in the United States and is fast becoming a worldwide health problem.

See where you fit in the following BMI scale. It's a fairly accurate way of determining whether you are overweight:

- 18–24 BMI: healthy
- 25–29 BMI: overweight
- 30–39 BMI: obese
- 40+ BMI: morbidly obese (dangerously overweight)

To learn how to calculate your BMI, talk with your doctor or visit the Centers for Disease Control website—www.cdc.gov/healthyweight/

assessing/bmi/index.html—to find a calculator for assessing your own BMI.

The Finnish Geriatric Intervention Study to Prevent Cognitive Impairment and Disability (FINGER) is one of the most important investigations on obesity, lifestyle, and Alzheimer's disease. Among the many significant findings of this large, long-term study (the findings of which we'll examine more closely in our lifestyle chapter) was that those who were obese in midlife were more than twice as likely to develop AD later, even when smokers or those who suffered from high blood pressure or high cholesterol were not included in the group. When obesity was added to the profile of those who had both high cholesterol and high blood pressure, the risk of developing Alzheimer's increased up to sixfold.[4]

In another 2007 study, Rachel Whitmer, PhD, senior research scientist at the Kaiser Permanente in Oakland, California, confirmed that both obesity and being overweight is associated with an increased risk of dementia, Alzheimer's disease, and vascular dementia (a related condition that we'll look at shortly), even in those who do not have diabetes or cardiovascular disease. It's interesting to note that Dr. Whitmer's study, which appeared in the journal *Current Alzheimer Research,* also found that weight loss later in life puts people at a greater risk.[5]

We know that once people start getting the dementia associated with AD, they lose weight. But that's not to say that weight loss is part of the reason they get AD; nor is it a reason not to lose a few pounds if you're over your recommended BMI or weight. Remember that obesity, metabolic syndrome, and type 2 diabetes all increase risk for future dementia.[6]

But perhaps the most intriguing finding by Kaiser Permanente was the significance of *where* fat was located. While BMI represents the total fat level in the body, those people whose fat tended to settle at waist level showed a 72 percent increase in risk for dementia development later on.

This risk factor is known as "central obesity" and can be measured by a skin-fold thickness test. "Central obesity increased risk of dementia more than three decades later," according to Whitmer's article in a 2007 issue of *Neurology*.[7]

It's important to have regular physicals to check blood sugar and glycosylated hemoglobin levels. If you tend to accumulate fat around your waist, ask your doctor to perform a skin-fold test for you to determine your risk factors. If your BMI puts you at risk, make a weight-loss goal, possibly with the help of a nutritionist. Exercise thirty minutes a day at least five days a week; reduce your sodium intake; eliminate processed foods, fast foods, and soda; and eat a healthy whole-food, plant-based diet or adopt a Mediterranean-style diet. More about that in our lifestyle chapter.

Stroke and Vascular Dementia

A stroke occurs when blood flow to part of the brain is interrupted and the lack of oxygen and nutrients cause brain cells to die. Damage to the body's blood vessel network starves the brain of oxygen and vital nutrients needed for cells to work properly. Nerve cells are particularly vulnerable. There are various ways this can happen.

Blocked arteries or blood clots are the most common cause of stroke, affecting seven hundred thousand Americans annually. Blood clots arise from inflamed arterial plaques and from an unhealthy heart. When blood clots break off and travel in the bloodstream to the brain, they can become lodged in an artery. If this happens, the area of the brain supplied by that artery will die.

Another cause of stroke is a ruptured blood vessel in the brain. This can result in what's known as a "cerebral hemorrhage," or bleeding within the brain. Uncontrolled hypertension (high blood pressure) is the most common cause of cerebral hemorrhage. Abnormalities in cerebral blood vessels, including aneurysms (a ballooning of the vessel wall) and arteriovenous malformations (an abnormal collection of blood vessels), can also produce bleeding in the brain. We all have a network of vessels known as our vascular or circulatory system. *Vascular* comes from a Latin word for "hollow container." Any condition that affects this system is considered vascular disease.[8] Diseases arise from problems with your arteries, veins, and vessels that affect how blood flows. A vascular disease can lead to our tissues not getting enough blood, a condition called ischemia, as well as other serious and even life-threatening problems.[9] If there is a blockage of the carotid arteries in your brain,[10] it can lead to a stroke or mini-stroke, which is called a transient ischemic attack (TIA).[11] Symptoms include weakness on one side of the body, vision problems, and slurred speech. These events are "transient," which means they can often resolve within twenty-four hours. Not all narrowing of blood vessels going to the brain leads to stroke. Stroke occurs only when the blood vessels are actually blocked or burst.

For more information on stroke warning signs, visit the American Stroke Association at www.stroke.org.

Vascular Dementia

Vascular dementia is considered the third leading cause of dementia in the United States, and it can occur separately from Alzheimer's disease, although there is considerable overlap. Vascular disease is caused by narrowing and blockage in blood vessels to the brain, a major contributor to vascular dementia and AD.

Some may remember when we used to call dementia and AD "hardening of the arteries." Well, evidence now suggests that there might have been some truth in that after all. So what is the risk of getting AD if one suffers from vascular disease? In a twenty-year study of nearly 1,500 people, published in the 2006 issue of *The Lancet Neurology*, researchers created a simple method for predicting the risk of late-life dementia in middle-aged people based on their medical profiles. They found there are several vascular risk factors associated with dementia, including older age, low education (people with higher education tend to take better care of themselves physically), hypertension, high cholesterol, and obesity. The bottom line is, these risk factors for vascular disease should be managed aggressively with your doctor by discussing lifestyle and dietary changes as well as medications that open blood-flow pathways.[12]

Heart Disease

Heart disease is a broad term that encompasses many health conditions, including:

- *Atherosclerosis.* Blockages and narrowing of the arteries of the heart that supply critical blood flow essential to its survival.
- *Valvular.* Narrowing and immobility of the valves in the heart.
- *Arrhythmia.* Irregular heart rhythm leading to inefficient heart pumping.
- *Congestive heart failure.* An inability to pump as efficiently as necessary to prevent blood flow from backing up into the lungs.
- *Cardiomyopathy.* Weakening and immobility of the walls of the heart, which are made out of muscle.

Heart Disease and Alzheimer's in ApoE Carriers

We discussed the role of the ApoE gene in lipid metabolism earlier. Several studies, including one conducted in 2011 by Mount Sinai School of Medicine and the Department of Psychiatry Brain Bank in New York City, showed the connection between the ApoE gene and heart disease. The discovery of the ApoE gene for Alzheimer's disease was made while doing a cardio lipid test. The researchers examined the hearts and brains of ninety-nine subjects who were devoid of cerebrovascular disease at the time of death. These scientists discovered that coronary artery disease, and to a lesser degree atherosclerosis, had significant links to the density of plaques and tangles in the subjects' brains. This link was especially strong among those with the ApoE allele. In other words, coronary artery disease contributes to the risk and extent of developing AD.[13]

It's important to watch for symptoms before diseases have progressed for too long. Frequently, by the time a patient sees a cardiologist or a neurologist, the symptoms are already too far down the path of coronary or Alzheimer's disease to stop or reverse the damage. Because hypertension is a risk of both heart disease and AD, you should keep a close eye on your blood pressure (BP).

The top number is the maximum pressure your heart exerts while beating (systolic), and the bottom number is the amount of pressure in your arteries between beats (diastolic). We start to worry when the systolic BP is consistently above 130. Your doctor may suggest reducing your salt intake, eating a heart-healthy diet, and being more physically active. Making these lifestyle changes is an important first step in treating high blood pressure.

Lowering your sodium intake (six grams or less of table salt), keeping your weight and body mass index (BMI) in the ideal range for your height, engaging in regular aerobic exercise, drinking less alcohol, and not smoking might be enough to control high blood pressure. Watch out for hidden sodium in processed foods by reading ingredient labels before you buy. If medication is indicated, ask your doctor about nitrendipine, which, as we just mentioned, is an effective antihypertensive drug that has been shown to reduce the rate of cardiac events in type 2 diabetic and hypertensive patients. Also, a calcium channel blocker (CCB) has shown to reduce the rates of stroke and cardiovascular events in elderly patients with isolated systolic hypertension (ISH). Diuretics that lower blood pressure by causing the kidneys to excrete more sodium and water are effective as well. By reducing fluid volume throughout the body, you can widen (dilate) your blood vessels. Blood pressure management, through diuretics and other medications, can reduce the risk of congestive heart failure by up to 75 percent.

Last word about BP and AD: in a 2017 report, the National Academies of Sciences, Engineering, and Medicine concluded that blood pressure management—as well as cognitive training and physical activity—may play a role in helping prevent cognitive decline and dementia, citing "encouraging although inconclusive" evidence.[14] As a scientist, I applaud their caution. Still, I don't think you need to wait for further research: if you're concerned about AD, adopting all those healthy behaviors, including blood pressure management, makes good sense for many reasons. We'll talk more about physical activity and cognitive training later.

Traumatic Brain Injury

New evidence is rapidly emerging about the connection between traumatic brain injury (TBI) as a risk factor for Alzheimer's dementia. TBI was initially called "punch-drunk syndrome" (*dementia pugilistica*) because it was believed to be associated with boxing. We now know that TBI can result from any repeated head injury during sports that produces mechanistic changes to the brain that could lead to the accumulation of tangles, chronic neuroinflammation, and nerve cell death.

Unlike mild repetitive head injuries, several epidemiological studies have shown that a single episode of a severe TBI is a major risk factor for AD, although more studies are needed to confirm this finding. Scientists are certain, however, that people with Alzheimer's dementia get it earlier and experience more extreme symptoms when there has been a head injury. Additionally, multiple blows to the head can stretch nerve fibers and cells, disrupting normal cellular function in the brain. It is possible that repeated blows to the head can result in microscopic strokes (microhemorrhages). This eventually leads to scarring in the brain and the disruption of brain chemistry itself. Similarly, military veterans who have suffered concussive blasts also have an increased risk for Alzheimer's dementia.

Because of heightened awareness, attention is now being paid by the sports industry and in the media about chronic traumatic brain injury (CTE), a neurodegenerative disease that damages the parts of the brain responsible for motor, cognition, and behavior. News reports about retired professional athletes who have been involved in tragic incidents, including suicide and murder, say CTE may have been the cause. To a far lesser extent, CTE can cause motor problems such as slurred speech; slow, uncoordinated movements; cognitive problems; and poor concentration. The CTE literature has spawned a debate among neurologists about whether plaques and tangles are created from the brain's response to the injury. Again, in CTE it's the repetition of the injury that causes impulsive behavior, lack of control, rage, forgetfulness. One of my patients was an NFL player who told me he often forgets to pick up his kids from school, despite his wife's text reminders.

CTE might not be progressive like Alzheimer's, but it can cause severe amnesia and aggressive behavior. You can have CTE as a result of a brain injury without it leading to Alzheimer's or dementia, but if you are an ApoE carrier and you have a head injury, evidence shows your dementia will progress at a much more accelerated rate.

Concussion is a mild form of traumatic brain injury (TBI) that usually happens after a blow to the head. And let's dispel a myth here: there is no evidence that a single concussion can cause AD, and it is a myth that if you fall asleep after being concussed, you will die. Symptoms include:

- Irritability
- Sensitivity to sound and light
- Headaches
- Lack of concentration and attention

- Memory loss
- Sleep disturbance

Currently, there are no reliable biomarkers of late-onset neurodegenerative diseases following TBI, because a definitive diagnosis can only be made via autopsy. Researchers are working on developing neuroimaging techniques, such as tau and amyloid positron emission tomography imaging, which would enable doctors to make an early diagnosis of CTE and provide interventions for possibly preventing AD following TBI.[15]

Sports such as football and soccer, where there is "heading" of the ball, have become controversial, with many parents forbidding their children from signing up for sports teams, and some soccer coaches not allowing "heading" for players under the age of eighteen, as young brains are especially vulnerable. If you or your kids are participating in sports or recreational activities where there is a danger of cranial impact, including cycling, skiing, horseback riding, ice hockey, lacrosse, rollerblading, and skateboarding, have them wear a helmet to protect those precious heads!

Smoking

Does anyone need just one more reason to quit smoking? If so, here's one: smoking can contribute to the onset of AD and even accelerate its development.

In 2004, I published a paper in the *Journal of Neurology* about a study that examined how chronic smoking affected the clinical and pathological features of Alzheimer's. My colleagues and I found that those individuals who were smoking cigarettes at the time of the onset of Alzheimer's tended to get the disease eight years earlier and were more likely to die of it eight years sooner as well. This effect was not driven by the presence of an ApoE gene, as we looked only at noncarriers of the allele. We measured the amount smoked in pack-years (the number of packs per day multiplied by the number of years smoked). Again, we found the more cigarettes smoked, the sooner the subject died. If the smoking ceased prior to the onset of Alzheimer's symptoms, then the prior smoking history had no effect on onset, duration, or outcome, and previous smokers were not different from nonsmokers in terms of their risk of AD. Our study did not support the idea that smoking protects the brain from Alzheimer's (and Parkinson's disease), as once believed, due to the delivery of nicotine, but instead it confirmed studies that found smoking contributes and even accelerates the development of Alzheimer's.[16]

Remember Rachel Whitmer, the scientist who conducted research on diabetes, vascular dementia, obesity, and AD at Kaiser Permanente in Oakland? In 2011, she participated in another study with colleagues about the neurological effects of smoking in midlife, concluding: "Heavy smoking in midlife was associated with a greater than 100% increase in risk of dementia, AD, and vascular disease more than two decades later. These results suggest that the brain is not immune to long-term consequences of heavy smoking."[17]

The very obvious thing that you can do here is to stop smoking. See the chapter on resources for support groups that will help you quit.

Depression

While depression strikes people of all ages, not surprisingly those with Alzheimer's are especially vulnerable. Depression can also be an early sign of dementia, emerging before memory loss.

As a member of the Alzheimer's Genetic Epidemiology group (MIRAGE), my colleagues and I examined nearly two thousand people with AD and more than two thousand of their unaffected relatives. We found a significant link between depressive symptoms and developing AD. Those diagnosed with Alzheimer's were more than twice as likely to have shown symptoms of depression in the year prior to diagnosis than were their relatives without dementia. Even more fascinating were the signs of depression early in life—up to twenty-five years before a diagnosis of Alzheimer's—which is a predictor of AD. This report led us to conclude that depression is a risk factor for later AD onset.

In Jamie's case, the causality was probably reversed. As you've read, learning that she was now a genetic time bomb plunged her into depression. How she finally came out of it, which is the subject of the next chapter, is a stirring reminder that this is another risk factor about which something can be done.

CHAPTER 9

Out of the Mouths
of B.A.B.E.S.

M y white 2009 Toyota Sienna was the kind of minivan you'd expect to see driven by a soccer mom. But having neither children nor a huge interest in soccer, I used it, instead, to haul flowers for many of my volunteer events up the mountains of Ramona and "down the hill," as we refer to it, into San Diego.

I called this van my Babemobile, and this particular sunny weekday morning, I was praying it would steer me down the road to sanity.

At this point, I was getting involved with the Alzheimer's Disease Research Center (ADRC). I was also learning more about the disease that I seemed fated to grapple with. Through my ongoing participation in the Banner study and as a now-sought-after voice for those who had been dealt a poor genetic hand, I felt like I was playing a small part in helping to combat AD as well.

Now, though, it was time to take care of myself.

My depression, my breakdowns, my fears—I could put them aside long enough to maintain composure when I spoke with an audience at an ADRC event or to the news media. But alone or at home, the depression would creep back, leaving me distraught and hopeless at times.

My braver and more competent former self seemed to have deserted me. Where was the young nurse who could coolly help stanch the bleeding of a brain shattered by a bullet? Where was the young woman who could stand up to an arrogant senior physician in order to advocate for a patient? The saleswoman with the confidence and moxie to close a major deal? The female marketing executive who jetted all over the Western US? I needed her back! I missed who I had been then.

Had all my former lives been a mirage?

By comparison, middle-aged Jamie couldn't even read a research paper without feeling anxious. I was still haunted by visions of the plaques in my brain spreading. Moreover, outside of Dr. Reiman and his colleagues, I was intimidated at the prospect of dealing with male medical authority, thanks to my experiences during the 2009 study.

I was frustrated. Even Doug's deep reservoir of patience was being tapped.

Doug had a friend at work, Dr. Marc Reeseman, a psychologist, who thought it might help if I talked to someone. He knew my story and understood that I needed a break from the mostly male-dominated world of medicine and scientific research I was becoming immersed in. He also understood that I needed a female therapist, and one who would show empathy for the kind of trauma I'd experienced. I didn't need someone else to tell me "just get over it and get on with your life," as if I'd been tackled in a football game and had to now get up, dust myself off, and go back in for the next play.

As crazy as it seems, that *is* the advice I'd heard from some friends: to get up and get on with life. I know that it was usually sincere and well-meant advice. And believe me, I wished I could have snapped my fingers and had everything back to the way it was before April 2009! That was back when my major health concern was my mysterious illness, maybe-MS, maybe-not-MS. Aside from some occasional weakness in my legs, those bodily symptoms were long gone. Now the pain, the fragility, the imbalance seemed to be not in my limbs or my gait but in my heart and my head, the result of this crazy and unexpected roller-coaster ride with a debilitating, frightening disease I didn't yet have and had barely thought about, before being unceremoniously informed that I was quite likely to become one of AD's victims.

At that point in my life, it occurred to me that I was suffering from a disease without actually having it! Who could possibly fix that? Dr. Adrianne Ahern.

Dr. Ahern was an author and a psychologist with a PhD operating a thriving practice near Del Mar. More importantly, she was a woman with a reputation of caring and compassion with her patients.

"I think you'll like her, Jamie," said Doug's friend Marc. "She's very kind."

That sounded good to me. I could use a little more kindness.

Dr. Ahern's office was in one of those nondescript office buildings, where you walk in and it's antiseptic and library-quiet but also anonymous. Each door is a different practice. Each door is closed. Initially, I was concerned. Would her style reflect the coolness of her space?

Not at all. When I walked into her office, the front desk staff was friendly, addressing me by name. I was offered water, encouraged to have a seat, and informed that I wouldn't be waiting long.

In a few minutes Dr. Ahern came out personally and ushered me into her office. It was small, intimate, welcoming. Its most impressive feature was a large, beautiful wooden bookcase, filled not with the textbooks and reference manuals that doctors usually display, but rather with books that everyday people have actually heard of or read. I saw some of Deepak Chopra's works, not to mention a copy of Dr. Ahern's own self-help book, *Back in Charge*.

I always notice a person's smile, and hers was radiant. With her brown, wavy hair and high heels, she looked polished and professional. She beckoned me to sit down in a rich, red leather chair facing her own black chair.

"It's nice to meet you, Jamie," she told me once we were seated. "So tell me, what brings you here today?"

While part of me wanted to pour out my heart to this woman I'd just met, I held back. Here she was, composed, successful, attractive. And here I was crazy, confused, ugly. Or at least that's how I felt. Insecure and inferior, not just compared to Dr. Ahern, but to everyone else in the world that wasn't born with a duplicate set of this stupid ApoE4 gene.

How could this apparent superwoman understand a defective piece of merchandise like me?

But since she had asked, I told her the story, an abbreviated version of the one you have read. To my surprise—because who would think a superwoman could be affected by mere words?—she appeared taken aback by what I had experienced. When I'd finished my tale of genetically induced woe, she asked me straight up: "Have you had thoughts about suicide, Jamie?"

There was no point in lying. "Yes," I said, shaking my head. "I have."

"Do you have a plan?"

"Yeah, pretty much. I was thinking pills, because I know I want to be a pretty corpse." She didn't laugh at my mild attempt at humor and continued to gauge my intentions.

"Well, how do you feel right now about that?"

"I'm not feeling that way right now," I said. "I mean, I have in the last few months, but today . . . at this moment . . . no."

"So what *are* you feeling right now?"

"I feel like I'm—like I'm falling into this abyss, and I won't be able to climb back out." I paused. "And I'm hoping you can throw me a life preserver."

Dr. Ahern, who invited me to call her by her first name, nodded thoughtfully. Then she looked me squarely in the eye. "It's clear to me that you've been through something traumatic, Jamie. But I think I can help you get through this. I think we can get you out of that abyss."

I wanted to hug her. Driving home that night, I felt better than I had in weeks. Dr. Ahern had validated my feelings. She acknowledged that I'd gone through a traumatic experience, and to me that alone seemed like a small victory. I'd been wondering if what I was feeling was all in my head. Whether I really was, as some had suggested, overreacting to a situation that I should simply accept as others had.

About six weeks into our sessions, she gave my feelings a name. "PTSD?" I exclaimed when Dr. Ahern told me. "I thought only people in the military got post-traumatic stress disorder."

"The definition has broadened," she said, explaining the new guidelines. "Essentially, it's a normal reaction to an abnormal situation."

Well, that much fit. I hadn't yet met anyone who thought my experience was anything but strange and anxiety provoking!

The doctor went on to explain that PTSD is now viewed by the mental health profession as something that can affect any person who has endured a traumatic experience, whether in the military or in civilian life. In the American Psychiatric Association's revised *Diagnostic and Statistical Manual of Mental Disorders* (DSM), PTSD is characterized by three sets of symptoms: reliving the event through intrusive memories and dreams, emotional avoidance such as steering clear of reminders of the trauma and detaching emotionally from others, and hyperarousal that causes sufferers to startle easily, sleep poorly and be on alert for potential threats. These problems must last for a month or more for someone to qualify for the PTSD label.

"And yes, you have some of the symptoms," Dr. Ahern told me.

I started reading more about PTSD, and in subsequent sessions the doctor explained it to me further. She pointed out, for example, my recurring, frightening dreams. The latest, which I had reported to her a few sessions earlier, were really scary. I was desperately trying to prevent attackers from coming through the door of my home. These unknown, faceless invaders were pounding, slicing, and hacking away, and I was trying unsuccessfully to stop them. I'd throw a punch, and it would land harmlessly. In another variation of that dream, I had been shot, and there was blood spurting from wounds in my chest. And yet I continued to flail away at my anonymous opponents. Sometimes in the dream, I'd hear myself saying, "Am I going to live; am I going to live?" Sometimes I'd wake up screaming.

Dr. Ahern helped me interpret those dreams. I eventually figured out that the invaders whose faces I never saw were those whose callous treatment of me in the wake of my 2009 test results had sparked this downward spiral. I had suffered an injustice, and I had been presented with a grim picture of a possible future. But I also came to realize during my sessions they weren't the only ones I was afraid of. It was Alzheimer's disease itself that, in my dreams, was trying to break through the sanctuary of my home, my life, and take me.

Yet, I kept fighting. Fighting for my life!

Soon, my anxiety began to lessen, and the dreams became less frequent. That was really a breakthrough for me. But I also sensed that I was now at a critical moment. I knew I wasn't nuts (or at least not completely!). Where should I go from here? A couple of distinct options emerged.

"I feel like I'm at a fork in the road, Adrianne." I now called my doctor by her first name.

"What do those roads look like?" she asked.

"Well, one of them is pretty dark." That route, I explained, could involve legal action against Dr. Leyland and his organization. And given how much attention was becoming focused on genetic disclosure in the years since I took the test, I suspected I might have a pretty good case too.

Adrianne frowned. "Ok, what's the other road like?"

"Something a little more positive."

I wasn't quite sure what that would be, but I sensed it would most likely mean mobilizing some of the skills and resources in order to get more involved in the fight, the fight against the other invader of my dreams: AD itself.

Adrianne listened.

"So basically Jamie, you've got a choice between a dark road and a bright road."

"Yeah, I suppose so."

"Which one would bring more joy to your life?"

Pausing a moment, Adrianne continued, "You know I can't tell you which one to take. But I know you well enough to know that it'll be the right road."

The right road. The *bright* road. And of course, she was correct, again.

Sure, I would have loved an apology and assurances that no one else would have to go through what I did, but that was already in the past. And given the fact that I regularly see commercials for genetic testing services on TV, I suspected plenty of people will continue to open PDFs or click on links and find disturbing genetic news, much of which will be presented to them completely out of context. I would urge them not to learn this vital information in that fashion, but I doubted that my getting one researcher in Southern California to admit that the way he'd treated this situation was wrong would change many minds.

Besides, what I really wanted was a lot more important than apologies for what happened in the past. It was time to start looking to the future.

Since my genetic skeletons had come tumbling out of the closet in 2009, I had learned much about the science and the scope of Alzheimer's. I saw more clearly than ever the breadth and depth of the epidemic, how it was affecting its victims and their families. As in the dream, there was a strong possibility that this faceless disease could be coming to get me before long. If so, I was determined to go down swinging.

I knew I still had the strength to do it. At last, the tenacity of Jamies in the past—the OR nurse, the saleswoman, the executive—seemed to come coursing back.

I'd learned from the experts at Banner and the ADRC that the way to combat this was through research—research that would eventually yield better treatments or preventive measures. My volunteer work at the ADRC and my participation in the research study at Banner were significant but small steps. But there was a lot more I could do. If I was serious about fighting back, it was time to ramp it up. I needed another weapon.

DOING IT MY WAY

I'd been around the ADRC long enough to know that, like most not-for-profit institutions, the lifeblood for maintaining the mission—in this case, to keep the research labs humming—was money.

Maybe I could help add to the flow.

I asked Mary Sundsmo, program director of the Alzheimer's Disease Research Center, if I could organize a fundraiser for the ADRC. She sighed. "Jamie, I'd love it if you could, but any fundraiser for us has to be done through the university." Say no more. Like any large organization, that meant guidelines and protocols would need to be followed, layers of approval and reams of red tape would have to be navigated through.

I wanted to raise funds my way. "Okay, so how about this? What if I start my own 501(c)(3)? That way I can raise the money and then donate it directly to you?"

Mary's eyes twinkled. "That might work."

"That way, instead of my organizing it here and having to jump through hoops and have someone else say, 'You can't have this or you can't have that,' I can just do it my way!"

"I know you'd do a great job, Jamie. But it's going to be a lot of work."

"Well worth it, if we can help you guys move one inch closer toward beating this disease."

Mary smiled. "It's going to be exciting to see what you come up with."

A stylish fundraiser is exactly what I had in mind. "I'm on it!" I said. "And oh, by the way," I added, noticing Mary's lovely coral-colored blouse, "You look really nice in that top!"

Coral. 501(c)(3). Research. AD. ADRC. Mary. Bright road. It was all swirling through my head as I got in the Babemobile to drive home.

A name. I needed a name for this new organization I was going to create. A name was key.

I found myself thinking about all the fun I'd had in my minivan with my fellow Babes—a group of about fifteen women from Ramona. We'd had many an enjoyable girls-night-out in the Babemobile. For one of our friend's seventieth birthday, we'd held the party in the minivan. We had festooned the whole interior with balloons. I pulled into her driveway, invited her in, and when she slid open the side door . . . surprise! Balloons and friends came pouring out.

Ah yes, the Babemobile.

And then I had it. I called my friend Lynn—one of the main Babes—and explained my idea of starting a nonprofit. "And I think I have the name too," I continued. "Ready?"

"What is it?"

"Beating Alzheimer's by Embracing Science—B.A.B.E.S. for short!"

"Wow, it's perfect! B.A.B.E.S.! I'm in!"

Everybody loved it—except for the attorney, Robert. He walked me through the process of setting up a corporation with a 501(c)(3) non-profit designation. As we were finishing up, he cleared his throat. "Just one thing," he said.

"What?"

"This name."

"What about it?"

"B.A.B.E.S.? That could be a flag for the IRS. They could think you're setting up a nonprofit that's really just an excuse for a bunch of women to go out and drink wine and solve the problems of the world."

"Robert, are you telling me the IRS is run by a bunch of sexist men? Because that's kind of what that sounds like."

Poor Robert was flustered. He's a good man, and he had my best interests at heart, but like a lot of good men, he sometimes didn't realize that what he was saying was inadvertently demeaning to women. He apologized.

"Don't worry. I know you didn't mean it that way. We may have some fun with the name and at our events. But the goal here is to raise money and awareness for the needs of research that might save a lot of lives someday. I'm serious about this, dead serious."

Later, I hired a female attorney to complete the legal process. She loved the name. Apparently, it took another babe to get the concept of B.A.B.E.S.

We were off and running!

B.A.B.E.S. AND BLING

We held our first fundraiser at a local winery. We called it "Adopt a Vine and Wine." For an extra donation, you could adopt a vine. Later, that person would be invited to help harvest the grapes.

With assistance from the Babes, all of whom eagerly pitched in—we call ourselves "the Babe Brigade"—I spent hours creating name tags, working with the winery, designing the certificates of adoption, and helping to promote the event. I hadn't felt that kind of joy in a long time. It seemed as if the darkness was lifting. Things were going in a positive way. I liked this bright path!

About fifty people attended Adopt a Vine and Wine, and B.A.B.E.S.

raised six thousand dollars. A respectable first event. Mary Sundsmo was there and was thrilled. "Gosh, what a nice debut," she said at the end. "I'm proud of you, Jamie."

For our second fundraising campaign, I had an idea: bracelets. The Babemobile and I paid a visit to a bead store, a wholesaler in San Diego. I went into the back area where they had various sample bracelets made up. The one that caught my eye had coral-colored sparkly beads—specially ordered from China—and Czech crystal. I remembered the coral blouse Mary had been wearing. Somehow it just seemed serendipitous.

"That's it!" I said to the owner of the store. "Can you make about five hundred for me?"

I told him my story and what we were using these bracelets for, and he cut the price in half.

We promoted the bracelets on our new website and through word of mouth. For a donation we'd give you a bracelet as a gift. We called it "Babe Bling." Everyone wanted one. One afternoon soon after we kicked off the campaign, I walked into the supermarket in town, and the teenage checkout girl saw my bracelet.

"I know about that," she said excitedly. "It's for Alzheimer's, right?"

"It sure is," I said, taking it off and handing it to her. "And now it's yours. Spread the word!"

Even Doug wanted in. "Can I be a Babe too?" he asked me one night.

"Doug, you're a guy."

He feigned insult. "Well, real men can be Babes, you know."

Actually, he had a point. While I was deliberately reaching out to women, we didn't want to exclude half the market. The successful breast cancer charities had gotten men involved in supporting their cause; we should too.

"You're right," I said, and handed him a bracelet. "I officially pronounce you a Babe."

"Oh boy," he said with a smile.

We eventually gave away more than five hundred bracelets in return for suggested donations, and it was tons of fun, but the campaign also taught me an important lesson. I knew B.A.B.E.S. was never going to compete with the major Alzheimer's groups, nor did we want to. If anything, we wanted to support all the good work being done by so many institutions. But if we were going to succeed, we had to be creative and imaginative. Babe Bling helped us stand out in the San Diego area—and even farther. Those little coral-colored trinkets would help usher me into the US Capitol in Washington, DC—and an entirely new aspect of my work with Alzheimer's.

HITTING ON ALL CYLINDERS

I sat up straight in my chair when I opened my inbox: there was an e-mail from Meryl Comer. Meryl is a big name in the world of Alzheimer's. A former broadcast journalist, she is president and CEO of the Geoffrey Beene Foundation Alzheimer's Initiative, and a board member of UsAgainstAlzheimer's, another major player in the AD advocacy arena. I'd contacted USA2—as they refer to themselves—some weeks earlier, letting them know about me and my B.A.B.E.S. and checking to see if there was any way we could work together.

Meryl was ready to take me up on that offer. In her e-mail she invited me to be a founding member of a new group, WomenAgainstAlzheimer's. High on their agenda would be an all-women's summit meeting in Washington to press the case for more funding with members of Congress.

I knew from my work at the ADRC that this was a big priority. AD was near the bottom of the list for research funding but was near the top for resources spent on treatment. It made no sense, a point Meryl has made eloquently in many interviews.

"We need to wage a war on Alzheimer's, just as we did with cancer," she told one senior living blog. "How can the government spend two hundred billion dollars annually on care and less than one percent on research? We need to be on the fast track for therapies, like HIV/AIDS and cancer."

My sentiments exactly. I told Meryl she could count me in. And so it was, a few months later, in May 2013, I found myself, along with thirty-seven other women representing other various Alzheimer's-related organizations around the country, at an event at The Phillips Collection in Washington, DC. We were the founding members of the new WomenAgainstAlzheimer's group, and we had come to Washington to petition members of Congress to increase funding for research on the disease.

The dinner, attended by about a hundred people, was our kickoff. Opened in 1921, The Phillips Collection was the country's first museum devoted to modern art. When we were gathered together for a group photo, we were reminded not to bump into any of the paintings. True, we were all in heels and maybe a little unsteady. This struck me as rather humorous. I thought to myself, *Just my luck that now would be the time when I lose my balance and go crashing into the wall.* I imagined the aftermath of that. "Oh, sorry, I put a big gash in that priceless Van Gogh! You can just fix that with some Krazy Glue, can't you?"

Fortunately, I and everyone else stayed upright. Afterward we had a wonderful dinner hosted by chairman George Vradenburg and his lovely cofounder wife, Trish.

I smiled at the woman next to me and introduced myself.

"I'm Annie Kuster," she replied. Actually, she was Rep. Annie Kuster, a congresswoman from New Hampshire. Annie seemed genuinely curious to know my story, and when I told her about myself and offered her some Babe Bling (of course I'd brought along a box of bracelets), she laughed. "These are really pretty!" she said.

I told her that I had a meeting scheduled the next day with Rep. Susan Davis, from a California district near mine. "Oh, I know Susan," Annie said. "She's one of my friends."

"Really?" I reached into my handbag and pulled out another bracelet. "Just in case you see her before I do, would you mind giving her some Babe Bling for me?"

Annie laughed. "I certainly will."

The next morning, we had our meetings scheduled. The newly formed WomenAgainstAlzheimer's was pressing to have the National Institutes of Health (NIH) allocate more money for AD research. In groups of three or four, we'd meet with the staff members of various members of Congress, briefly tell our story, and make the case for increased funding. My pitch was simple: I told them about my genetic risk and suggested that if we didn't increase funding to help find a cure, I could soon be one of the disease's victims.

The look on the faces of the often-jaded congressional staffers—used to having special pleaders in their office on a daily basis—suggested that my story had an effect.

Our efforts, along with those of other organizations, worked: the NIH funding for AD research has increased every year since 2013.

My last appointment of the day was with Representative Davis. By that time, I'd been on my feet for hours traipsing around the Capitol and they were sore. As we say in Ramona, my dogs were barking. But I still had Babe Bling to sling and an important message to deliver.

I met with one of Representative Davis's staffers, a young man who looked like he could have been the son I never had. He listened, was quite clearly moved by what I told him, and promised me he would discuss it with his boss. "I know she cares about this issue," the young man said. "I'll make sure she gets the information." I gave him some bling for his girlfriend. "Or your mom," I said, as he blushed.

We shook hands, and as I walked out of the office and turned the corner down the hall, there was Representative Davis herself, whose face I'd seen in the papers back home, walking toward me as she returned from another meeting.

"Hi," I said. "You must be Susan Davis."

She studied me for a second, and then burst out, "You're the one with the bracelets!"

Mentally, I thanked Annie Kuster. "Yes, I am," I said. "And I'd like to tell you a little more about what we need to do to fight Alzheimer's."

Susan promised to meet with me one-on-one when we were both back in San Diego, and she was as good as her word. Not only did we meet, but Representative Davis subsequently attended some of our B.A.B.E.S. fundraisers, sporting an official B.A.B.E.S. bracelet on her wrist when she arrived.

After the summit and my subsequent meetings with Susan, I sensed that my role and that of B.A.B.E.S. was shifting. Yes, we were and still remain an organization committed to fundraising for Alzheimer's research. But, along with my Babe Bling, I began to recognize that my story and my unusual 4/4 status commanded attention in the AD world. I suppose my sales background didn't hurt either. I began to realize that I could possibly do as much as a national advocate for Alzheimer's research as I could do through our local fundraisers.

I was also hugely impressed with the people behind UsAgainstAlzheimer's, Meryl Comer and George and Trish Vradenburg. Like most of those involved in this cause, they'd all watched loved ones suffer with AD. Trish, who had had a long and successful career as a television writer before sadly dying from a heart attack in 2017, wrote a play, *Surviving Grace*, about dealing with her mother's struggles with AD. We saw a reading of it in Washington, DC, and I thought it really captured the frustrations and heartbreak of the disease from the perspective of a caregiver.

I suggested to George, Trish, and Meryl that we bring *Surviving*

Grace out West. "We'll do it as a joint collaboration between B.A.B.E.S. and WomenAgainstAlzheimer's," I said. Meryl, who had asked me to be her eyes and ears for the organization on the West Coast, was enthusiastic. "Let's do it!" she said.

Now while I would love to add "Executive Producer" to my résumé, I have to be honest—*they* did most of the work. An event team flew out to San Diego, found the venue—the Joan B. Kroc Theater—as well as celebrity readers, and did most all the other groundwork.

The cast was superb: actress Marilu Henner was a reader, as was former NPR host Diane Rehm. We sold out the theater, and everyone seemed to enjoy the show. I was thrilled when philanthropist Darlene Shiley—who was also a reader and is the woman for whom the Shiley-Marcos Alzheimer's Disease Research Center is named—attended and gave a very generous donation to the ADRC.

My biggest contribution to the San Diego production of *Surviving Grace* was the presence of one of the other star readers. Through a friend of mine, Carolyn Olsen, we were able to get singer Helen Reddy to participate. As I sat in the audience that night, listening to the woman whose number one hit "I Am Woman" had been an early feminist anthem in the 1970s, I couldn't help but think that I was roaring, too, and not out of the same pain and despair as I had been in the months and years after learning my AD risk.

Like the Babemobile that had served me well, I felt as if I was finally hitting on all cylinders. And while the road ahead might be uncertain, I was enjoying the ride.

CHAPTER 10

Becoming a Caregiver

M entally, I tried to rehearse my words as I approached the manager of the Sprouts natural food supermarket in Rancho Bernardo.

"Hi, just want to let you know, my dad's a shoplifter." *No, no, no. He'll be dialing 9–1–1. I need something better.* "Hi, how are you? That older man with the white mustache in the candy aisle? He's trying to rob you blind. But it's not his fault." *Scratch.*

Eventually I came up with the right language. "Hi, how are you? I just want to let you know that my dad has Alzheimer's, and he sometimes puts things in his pocket and forgets to pay for them. But don't worry, I'll make sure we pay for everything."

Ah, the joys of caregiving for an AD patient.

I told some of my family members about this incident, and we all had a good laugh. But the funny moments for a caregiver are few and far between, as I learned after my dad was diagnosed with AD in 2008, the year before I learned about my own 4/4 status.

When my father was in his early seventies, Jane—who was his wife for thirty years after he and Mom had divorced—shared her concerns with me about my dad's confused behavior. At the time, I didn't want to tell her what I knew in my heart: he was showing signs of AD. Jane took him to his primary care provider, who diagnosed him with depression and prescribed an antidepressant. I was pleased with this diagnosis, although at the time I had no clue that depression can be one of the first changes seen in those with AD.

But my father's cognition continued to decline, and he started getting lost while driving, another telltale symptom of Alzheimer's. Jane's first solution was to sit in the passenger seat and guide him along the route so he could feel as though he was still in control. But soon he was evaluated by a geriatric neurologist who confirmed my fears that Dad was in the early stages of AD. The doctor said he could no longer drive and contacted the DMV to have his license revoked. My dad, then 77, was furious. Jane loved my father dearly and did everything she could to keep him at home, but it became increasingly difficult for her to live with his outbursts and erratic behavior.

At the time he started showing signs, my own emotions were in free fall after hearing the news about my 4/4 status and the likelihood of my getting AD, so I was grateful that Jane, along with her grown daughter Cathy, had taken on the daily caregiving responsibilities, which were both physically and mentally taxing. While they took the brunt of the burden for my father's care, they would include me as part of the decision-making process. It was so heartbreaking going to the doctors' appointments with them, knowing what the end would be like.

Jane, Cathy, and I were all stressed, conflicted, and angry about what was happening to my dad. It is not uncommon for families to get pulled apart, especially when there is disagreement about what should be done at the end of life and who should be in charge of making those difficult decisions.

While Jane and I saw eye to eye on most things concerning my dad's care, there were times when I found myself so angry with my dad for what I perceived as his irascible or stubborn behavior. Eventually, I learned that this is another common theme among children or spouses involved in caregiving for patients of AD. I was reacting to memories of my father, Lawton Henry TenNapel, and the way he had been forty years in the past, when he was an often-angry, insensitive parent. But this was no longer the man who had popped my broken shoulder in place and told me to stop whining. This was a man with plaques and tangles that had strangled his brain, a man who was no longer responsible for his own behavior.

My anger toward him gave way to pity.

When I accompanied the CNN crew to interview Dad and Jane at their house for the documentary on Alzheimer's, I lost it. The crew rang the doorbell, and I crouched against the door, sobbing. My mind screamed, *I can't do this!* The camera crew had to give me a moment to pull myself together. A geyser of emotions about "coming out" as an ApoE4 carrier and the fact that my father's disease was going to be documented for the world to see prompted the meltdown.

But I knew I needed to pull it together for my family and for the cause. CNN got the footage they needed, but I wept every time I watched the scene in the documentary where I interacted with my father. I cried because he was now a weak and vulnerable man, and also because I knew I'd never have the chance to tell him how afraid I had been of him at times growing up. But more importantly, I cried because he'd never be able to understand how much I loved him despite that.

After that I tried to help Dad recover some of the little things he'd enjoyed in life as a younger man, before Alzheimer's extinguished his spark. I remembered that when I was a child, he had a ritual when he got home from work: he would grab a cold beer from the fridge to help him relax after another strenuous day driving his tractor trailer. It was usually a Coors—none of those fancy microbrews of today. He'd just have one, enough to wet his whistle, but he truly enjoyed that end-of-the-day ritual.

FIGHTING FOR MY LIFE

Now, the care facility he was in would not allow alcohol, for obvious reasons. But I wanted Dad to have some joy during this dreary, unforgiving time of his life. So on my way to visit him, I'd stop at the supermarket and buy him a six-pack of nonalcoholic beer. It tasted like regular beer, and he had no idea that it was zero proof. These "beer runs" brought him back to happier times.

One day Dad begged me to take him with me when I went on a beer run. He was having a good day so I agreed, totally forgetting that, as Jane had warned me, he had started shoplifting as his Alzheimer's progressed. Once we got to the store, he ignored the selection of beers and made a beeline to the candy section, helping himself to as many loose candies—chocolate covered nuts and raisins—as he could fit in his pockets. I was mortified! I tried handing him a plastic bag to capture what he was taking, so I could pay the cashier, but he would have none of it. He wanted to carry his loot home in his pockets.

"Dad," I said, exasperated, and embarrassed. "You can't steal!"

"Oh, yes I can," he snapped. "Go away!"

There was no stopping this geriatric kleptomaniac! I mustered up the courage to walk over to the service desk and find the store manager. He was average height with salt-and-pepper gray hair, and he flashed an understanding grin when I told him. "It's okay," the manager said. "We know your father, and that's what we call 'sampling.'"

What a beautiful lesson I learned that day. Sometimes, bringing Alzheimer's out of the shadows gives people the opportunity to be kind and understanding. The disease was also teaching me how to love my father again. When I looked into his eyes, I could see my own reflection and my own destiny staring me in the face. How could I not feel love for a man who was so weak and broken?

When my father was dying, I called my siblings to let them know. They couldn't come because they lived too far away. Jane couldn't be there either, because it was too much for her emotionally, and she wanted to remember him as he was. I understood this. Each person handles death differently, and she just couldn't do it.

In the final hours, Jane's daughter Cathy went over to her house so she wouldn't be alone. Doug and I were at my father's bedside at the facility he had been living in. It turned out to be a profound moment. I will never question that there is life after death because of what I experienced on July 6, 2011, the day my father died.

That afternoon Dad was pale, and his breathing was labored and sporadic. I gently stroked his arm as soothing classical music played in the background, and I sponged his mouth to keep him comfortable. He had not been responsive for the previous twenty-four hours, and we knew he didn't have long to go. Shortly after Dad's breathing and heartbeat ceased, and he'd officially been pronounced dead, Doug left the room to start making calls to the family.

I sat there for a while with his body and the hospice nurse, an extremely intuitive and spiritual woman. "Your dad is having a hard time leaving," she told me.

"What do you mean?" I asked, completely confused at first. "Why?"

"He's worried about Jane," she told me. I pondered this. My dad had been physically dead for at least ten minutes by this point. He couldn't possibly hear anything now, couldn't possibly be worrying about Jane or me or anyone—could he?

After a moment, I decided to take this nurse at her word, and I walked over to Dad, leaned in, and whispered in his ear. "Dad, Jane is fine," I told him. "She wanted to remember you as you were. She's with Cathy."

At that moment, I felt a sudden rush of energy coming from his body through my heart. I truly believe that at that moment I felt his soul leaving this earth. I turned to the nurse and she sensed it too.

"He's gone," she said.

Happily, our family came together for Dad's memorial service. Jane and Cathy chose a wonderful venue, and my sister Cindi, who has a degree in religious studies, gave a beautiful sermon. Everyone spoke about our favorite, fun moments with our father, which peppered that solemn occasion with lighthearted moments.

But it had been a long and trying three years since his diagnosis. I reflect upon that time in my life daily and send up a prayer for the many caregivers still in the midst of their own fight with AD.

THE ROAD TO CAREGIVING

More than fifteen million family caregivers help someone with Alzheimer's disease or other dementia, according to the Alzheimer's Association. Perhaps you are one too—or about to become one. If so, I want to share the wisdom I have learned from my experience as a caregiver, from the Alzheimer's community, and from my faith.

Taking care of someone with Alzheimer's requires all the energy, empathy, and patience you can muster. Every AD caregiver I know needs encouragement and inspiration. While caregivers are generous with their time, energy, and love, burnout is a struggle for many. If you are experiencing caregiver fatigue, do not despair. Studies show that 30 to 40 percent of dementia caregivers suffer from depression and emotional stress, and 40 percent of Alzheimer's caregivers die *before* the patient, due to the physical and emotional strain of caregiving.[1] There are many resources to help you manage caregiver stress.

Actor Gene Wilder, who was famous for his roles in *The Producers*, *Willy Wonka and the Chocolate Factory*, and *Young Frankenstein*, was diagnosed with Alzheimer's in 2013. His wife, Karen Wilder, wrote an essay for *Guideposts* magazine about how the disease not only took control of his life, but of hers as well. "In addition to destroying—piece by piece—the one who's stricken with [Alzheimer's], it ravages the life of the person caring for its victims," Karen wrote. "In our case, I was that person."[2] Gene Wilder passed away in August 2016 with Karen by his side until the very end.

PREPARING FOR AD

Both caregivers and AD patients need time to adjust to the diagnosis and to plan ahead for the future. Here, and in every phase of the caregiving process, the Family Caregiver Alliance (FCA) is an excellent source of information—a nonprofit organization that supports family and friend caregivers.

The FCA offers these tips for dealing with the early stages of AD:

- *Learn as much as you can about the disease.* The more you know about AD, the more prepared you will be as a caregiver. I hope reading our book has been a helpful part of your AD education. And of course, as the knowledge base is constantly changing, stay abreast with the latest developments, and don't be afraid to ask your physician.

- *Take it one step at a time.* Yes, AD is a progressive disease. But don't worry about what's coming. Start with the early and middle stages of the disease first, and worry about the late stage later. Taking it a step at a time will keep you from feeling overwhelmed. One of the most difficult things to learn as a caregiver is to differentiate between the disease and your loved one, especially in the early stages. You might find yourself thinking, *He's doing this to spite me!*, or, *She is just being lazy.* In these cases, the disturbing behavior is usually caused by the disease and not an attempt by the person with AD to hurt or frustrate the caregiver. It was so painful for me to watch my father going through the stages of AD, but it was also helpful to remind myself that his behavior was the disease and not him.

- *Get emotional support.* Finding other caregivers to talk with is one of the best ways to learn about and process your own experience. You will also need emotional support, so seek help from counseling, therapy, support groups, friends, and family members. The goal is to create a go-to team you can call on anytime during your AD journey.

- *Changing roles.* Losing the ability to drive is a familiar symptom of AD, so caregivers must prepare for this eventuality by being prepared to take over the driving (as Jane did in the case of my father), or recruiting volunteer drivers from family and friends, using public transportation, or car services. If the person with AD used to cook family meals, the responsibility will shift to the caregiver, who must learn how to cook or make alternative arrangements through food delivery (if affordable). There are many prepared food services from the high-end Blue Apron to God's Love We Deliver and Meals on Wheels. Similarly, if the person with AD was once in charge of finances, you might have to assume this role or assign this task to someone in the family or to a trusted accountant. Sort out these new roles and divisions of labor early so you won't be left scrambling when the time comes.

- *Cost.* All serious illnesses are expensive, but AD is especially so because it can linger for many years. It is advisable, therefore, to begin developing strategies for the financial demands that will likely be placed on the family as the disease progresses. My Grandma Ethel, Great-Grandma Neva's daughter, was lucky to have a pension and social security to help pay expenses when she had AD, but unless one has a large nest egg in the form of an IRA, 401k, or other retirement savings, families can go bankrupt from medical expenses. Make sure to review your insurance coverage, including health, disability, and long-term care. Unfortunately, Medicare does not pay for long-term care or custodial care, so you will have to supplement these costs—but Medicare does pay for hospice care. Medicaid, the safety net for those living on a limited income, does provide coverage for those who qualify. Free health insurance counseling is also available to seniors. To locate help in your community, go to www.eldercare.gov.

- *Legal advice.* Eldercare lawyers can be extremely helpful when making medical, financial, and even personal decisions for those with AD. It's a good idea to do the legal paperwork as early as possible in the disease process, even prior to a diagnosis. If you wait too long, the patient might be considered unable to sign legal documents. "A Power of Attorney for Finances and Power of Attorney for Healthcare (Advanced Health Care Directive) can ensure that the person with AD is cared for by trusted family members or friends," the FCA advises. "Without these documents, caregivers may have to petition for conservatorship through court proceedings in order to obtain the right to make decisions on behalf of the person with AD. The family may also lose access to bank accounts if a member is not co-named on the account(s)." Having a completed and signed will and trust is also imperative and keeps heirs from fighting amongst themselves. Be sure those with AD sign a Do Not Resuscitate (DNR) form while they are still of sound mind, if that's their wish. Not having this end-of-life discussion can create enormous confusion and heartache for a family. Free and low-cost legal services are available to seniors, and the resources section at the end of this book gives more information about organizations that can help with legal issues.[3]

Have more questions about caregiving? Don't be afraid to talk with your doctor.

In addition to taking on the household chores, shopping, transportation, and personal care, caregivers are often responsible for administering medications, injections, and other medical treatments. I'm a former nurse, so I am trained to do this, but for most caregivers this is new, and there will be a learning curve. This is where your relationship with the doctor and health-care staff come into play. Don't be afraid to ask questions, and make sure you write those questions down as they come up, and keep good notes on medications and other observations of your loved one's symptoms.

While you're at it, don't forget or ignore your own health-care needs, as many caregivers suffer from debilitating physical and psychological stress as they become focused on their charge. Building a partnership with the attending physician to address the health of both the patient and you, the caregiver, is essential. It will ultimately be your responsibility to communicate with the health-care professionals to ensure that everyone's needs are met, including your own.

MOVING DAY: HELP WITH THE TRANSITION

One of the hardest parts of being a caregiver is making that decision to move your loved one to a facility that is equipped to care for people with AD. Find out if there is a memory care section that specializes in dementia and related illnesses. Neither Great-Grandma Neva, my Grandmother Ethel, nor my father wanted to leave their homes, which is completely understandable, and frequently the patient will flatly refuse and end up going kicking and screaming (literally). This is why planning ahead is so important, because it can help reduce the fear of the unfamiliar and ease the transition for all involved. Here are some tips from the Mayo Clinic and from me to help you prepare for moving day.

Have a Conversation about Moving

Try talking to your loved ones while they are still able to make reasonable choices about the kind of living arrangements they prefer (roommate, no roommate, a faith-based facility, city or country setting, and so on). This will take the guesswork out of what the patient might want. Make frequent visits to the residence at different times of day before you decide. Speak with the staff, including the social worker in charge of patients and setting up a care team, about your loved one's background and any special needs. Provide as much detail as possible on your family member's medical and mental health history, including a complete medication list.

If possible, include the patient in these visits, though I realize this might not be a good idea if he or she is adamantly against moving, which can create more stress. But if the patient is willing, it can certainly help reduce anxiety to explore the new surroundings before moving in.

Bring Personal Items for the Room

Bring as many personal items as possible to make the room look and feel more familiar. Decorate with family photos and treasured items such as gifts from children and grandchildren; bring a favorite chair, quilt, or painting. According to the Mayo Clinic, "These belongings can trigger feelings of connectedness and ownership, as well as boost your loved one's sense of security." Label the pictures to help staff members, visitors, and patient identify the people in the photos, and spark conversations about the past. Be careful with heirlooms and priceless or irreplaceable items. There are digital frames that can be loaded with many photos that change every few minutes, if space is a factor. Consider bringing items that can be replaced easily if need-be, such as costume jewelry or copies of old photographs rather than originals. I hand tinted a copy of a photo of my father with his beloved dog, Dodo, that went with him wherever he was residing. He forgot many things, but he always remembered Dodo. Dodo was with him, even on the day he passed.[4]

There are several studies about the benefits of "reminiscence therapy" and how it taps into long-term memory and enables the AD patient to go back in time. When I use this technique with a friend of mine, she always brightens up and engages in conversation. It lasts a few hours and it makes my heart sing to see her perk up.

Stay in Touch

Leaving your loved one in the new home or facility might simultaneously bring on feelings of grief, loss, guilt, and, yes, even relief. These emotions are all normal. In the interest of self-care, make sure you have someone to support you on moving day. Call on a friend, family member, therapist, social worker, or support group. It might take a few months for the patient to become acclimated to his or her new living arrangement. Visit as often as you can, especially in the beginning, and encourage others to do the same.[5]

With time and patience most settle in eventually. This is what reportedly happened to Sandra Day O'Connor's husband, John, who suffered from Alzheimer's. After she stepped down as the first female justice on the US Supreme Court to care for him, she never imagined that he would fall in love with another woman. Yet, instead of feeling jealous, his wife of fifty-five years said she was "thrilled" with their romance, and relieved that the seventy-seven-year-old, who had become depressed and introverted, barely recognizing his own family, had found happiness in a new relationship with a fellow patient in his care home.[6]

An anecdote from my own family might also help here: my Grandmother Ethel was not at all happy about going to a facility. However, two months later, she met another resident, a kind gentleman named Orville who was around her age and in the early stages of dementia. Orville became her boyfriend. We all breathed a collective sigh of relief, knowing she would be fine, at least for the time being. It was lovely to see the two of them holding hands and cuddling like puppies. Grandma Ethel was happy in this new setting, and she had settled into her new home.

May your loved one be fortunate enough to find his or her Orville—or at least a peer that they can relate to.

COMMUNICATING WITH THE HEALTH-CARE TEAM

Remember, when it comes to AD care, it takes a team. Frequently the doctor at a facility only sees the patient for a few minutes, so make sure that he or she is made aware of your concerns, and don't be afraid to call on the health-care team (nurse, social worker, volunteer staff) for advice.

- *Prepare your questions in advance.* Make a list of your most important concerns and problems, and bring them with you to office visits or when the doctors make rounds. You will probably want to discuss changes in symptoms, medications, or general health of the care recipient, your own caregiving needs, and where you can get help to provide appropriate care.
- *Ask the nurse.* As a nurse, I know firsthand that many patients and caregivers can be intimidated by doctors, so don't hesitate to ask the nurses questions about anything you don't understand. In particular, the nurse can answer questions about various tests and examinations, preparing for surgical procedures, providing personal care, and managing medications at home.
- *Take someone else along with you to appointments.* A friend or family member not only lends support and comfort but can ask questions you may forget or feel uncomfortable asking. This person

can also take notes so that you remember what the physician or nurse has said. I can't tell you how much it helped Jane to know that I was there for support when she needed help in making those all-important decisions about my dad's care.

- *Try to make appointments in the morning or after lunch, which have the shortest waiting times.* Let the front desk know the reason for your visit before coming in so there is enough time for all your needs to be met. Call ahead to see if the doctor is behind schedule to reduce your wait time. You can also tell the receptionist if there are any special needs when you arrive.[7]

STEPS FOR MANAGING YOUR OWN STRESS

You cannot underestimate how stressful it is being a caregiver and how it can negatively impact your own health. Pay attention to early warning signs. For me, it was irritability, sleep problems, and forgetfulness, which turned out to be anxiety-provoked and not AD, which I feared. Once you recognize your own warning signs, take action to address your symptoms. Don't wait until you are calling 911 for yourself! Here's how:

- *Identify the source of your stress.* Ask, "What is causing me to feel so anxious?" Sources of stress might include feeling overwhelmed by what you need to do, family disagreements, questioning your ability to handle the situation, feelings of inadequacy, or not knowing when to say, "No, this is too much!"
- *Stay active and proactive.* Here I can speak from my experience as someone with a high risk for AD, as well as a caregiver. After finding out my genetic status, I was debilitated by my depression, which left me emotionally and even physically stunted. It was only by taking action to reduce my stress through therapy, research,

and action that I regained a sense of control. I also exercise when I can, and I want to do more. I know not everyone enjoys exercise, but you can significantly reduce your stress by doing even simple activities like taking nature walks, yoga and meditation, gardening, or having coffee or wine with a friend. Identify some stress reducers that work for you—and just do it!

- *Accept what you can and cannot change.* Borrowing from Al-Anon, keep in mind that we can only change ourselves; we cannot change another person. When you try to change things over which you have no control, you will only increase your sense of frustration. Ask yourself, "What do I have some control over? What can I change?" Even a small change can make a big difference. Here, you might be comforted, as I am, by the words taken from the original Serenity Prayer, attributed to American theologian Reinhold Niebuhr: "God grant me the serenity to accept the things I cannot change, the courage to change the things I can, and (the) wisdom to know the difference."[8]

Finally, another old saying bears repeating: you must save yourself before you can save others. Only when we help ourselves can we effectively help others. When your needs are taken care of, the person you care for will benefit too. It is not selfish or weak to exercise self-care. In fact, it's critical that you do so. Not only will adopting a healthy lifestyle help you be a better caregiver, recent evidence suggests that it can also help you reduce the risk of developing AD yourself, an important topic which Marwan explores in the next chapter.

CHAPTER 11

Protecting Yourself Against AD, Part One: Diet

MARWAN SABBAGH, MD

E ven though we researchers are looking for ways to prevent AD and to ultimately find a cure, it is potentially misleading to talk about prevention, which is not yet proven to be achievable. Rather, I'm going to refer to what we know will help protect you against dementia and AD or delay its onset.

So let's discuss what science has found to be the best steps to slow down the progression of the disease. Multiple studies have shown that lifestyle is key. If you or someone you know is at risk of getting AD (whether or not you or they have ApoE4), don't sit around passively waiting for the disease to take hold. Living a full, healthy, physically active lifestyle filled with nutritious food, close friends, and mental stimulation is the best thing you can do. And watching your weight and bad cholesterol can also help you stay as sharp as possible for as long as possible. Yes, there is something you can do, as the intervention studies and protocols found in Appendix 2 clearly show.

DON'T WAIT TO MAKE LIFESTYLE CHANGES

These are the steps you can take to help slow down the onset of AD and dementia. Because AD can start in the brain decades before symptoms appear, start following these steps as early as possible, even in your twenties or thirties. After all, each piece of the advice mentioned below can improve anyone's brain and physical health!

Eat a Brain-Healthy Diet

What you eat does more than affect your waistline—it affects your brain. As the Finnish Geriatric Intervention Study to Prevent Cognitive Impairment and Disability (FINGER) test, conducted by the Alzheimer's Research and Prevention Foundation, and other studies prove, diet ranks among the top lifestyle factors that will determine our ability to protect against Alzheimer's. (See more about the FINGER test in appendix 2.) Even taking risk factors into account, one of the most effective ways to fight or delay the onset of Alzheimer's is to retool a poor diet.

That's right. Eating better might help your brain work better and might ultimately stave off dementia and AD. The North American Aging Project recommends the Mediterranean diet, which I like, and other research suggests the whole food, plant-based diet (WFPB) is beneficial for the body and brain. Some like the ketogenic diet, which is controversial but has shown to help reduce symptoms of dementia and is likely best suited for the dementia state. But adhering to that diet is not fully proven. In fact, there are no diets with irrefutable data to recommend one above all others.

There is strong scientific evidence, however, that higher dietary intake of specific foods, such as those rich in the B-complex vitamins (especially B6, B12, and folates), antioxidants, anti-inflammatories, and unsaturated fatty acids will lower the risk of developing Alzheimer's. Many of the foods already in your kitchen can be your front line of defense against dementia and cognitive decline. If you're eating a standard American diet (aka SAD) and your fridge and freezer are filled with soda, processed, fried, and sugar-laden products, replacing them with fresh, nutrient-rich foods will help you combat cardiovascular disease, diabetes, obesity, cancer, and a myriad of illnesses, many of which are directly linked to Alzheimer's.

The Mediterranean Diet. This diet is modeled after what is eaten in countries such as Greece and Italy, which includes a variety of fresh fruits and vegetables, whole grains, nuts, fish, and little or no red meat or dairy products. The more colorful your meal, the healthier it is. So eat like an artist and your plate is your palette! One of the reasons this diet is so good for us is that it is lower in saturated fats (the bad fat) and higher in levels of good fats, such as those monounsaturated and polyunsaturated fatty acids found in fish, nuts, and olive oil.

Allow me to put a figurative underline and exclamation point next to the last item on that list. Recent research from Temple University suggests that EVOO (extra-virgin olive oil) can protect against memory loss, preserves the ability to learn, and reduces conditions associated with Alzheimer's disease. For those reasons (not to mention the fact that it's a delicious complement to many foods), I'm a big fan of EVOO—and you should be too!

As for the Mediterranean diet as a whole, here's some proof as to its effectiveness. Researchers based in New York City tracked more than 2,200 people without dementia for up to thirteen years, with an average tracking time of four years. They gave each participant a Mediterranean diet score ranging from zero to nine. Beyond slowing the development of Alzheimer's, adherence to the Mediterranean diet seemed to provide a link to a slower rate of cognitive decline, even after scientists adjusted for age, gender, ethnicity, education, caloric intake, BMI, and ApoE genotype. A follow-up of the study a few years later found that the higher the adherence to the Med diet, the lower the risk for AD, with the top one-third of subjects who continued to follow the diet having a 68 percent lower risk of developing Alzheimer's, compared with the bottom third who went off it.[1]

Similarly, a 2015 Rush University–Chicago study found that the MIND diet, a hybrid of the Mediterranean and the similar Dietary Approaches to Stop Hypertension (DASH) diet, consisting of fruits, veggies, whole grains, nuts, fish, and low-fat dairy products, was associated with slower cognitive decline. In this longer-range study, researchers investigated the diet–AD relationship in 923 participants, ages 58 to 98, for an average of 4.5 years. The results were assessed by subjects who self-reported via a food-frequency questionnaire. Those who followed the MIND diet had the lowest scores for AD.[2]

The Whole Food, Plant-Based Diet (WFPB). Another highly recommended brain-boosting diet is one filled with whole foods (unprocessed, unrefined, high fiber, low sugar) and plants (green, leafy vegetables). The concept of "whole" foods is this: eat plant-based foods in forms that are as close to their natural state as possible. Restaurants and other foodies like to call this farm-to-table foods. In other words, the closer the source of the food you consume and the less it is altered by chemicals and additives, the healthier it is for your body. Eat a variety of vegetables, fruits, raw nuts, seeds, beans, and legumes, and avoid salt, vegetable oil, and sugar. The aim is to get 80 percent of your calories from carbohydrates, 10 percent from fats, and 10 percent from protein. That's the WFPB short list. WFPB diets have been shown to robustly reduce cardiovascular disease. Studies are currently underway to determine if they have benefit in AD.

The Ketogenic Diet. The "keto" is high-fat, low-carb diet (think Perlmutter's Grain Brain and Atkins), in which the body produces ketones in the liver that are used as energy. Here's how it works: When you eat something high in carbs, your body will produce glucose and insulin. Glucose is the easiest molecule for your body to convert into energy. Because the glucose is being used as a primary energy source, your fats are not needed and are therefore stored. By lowering the intake of carbs, the body is induced into a state known as "ketosis." Ketosis is a natural process the body initiates to help us survive when food intake is low. During this state, we produce ketones, which are produced from the breakdown of fats in the liver. By overloading the body with fats and taking away carbohydrates, the body will burn ketones as the primary energy source. Optimal ketone levels are said to improve health, promote weight loss, and have physical and mental performance benefits.

In short, the ketogenic diet provides an alternative fuel for the brain. But alternative fuel may only be effective at certain stages of the disease, so it remains to be seen if the keto diet should be used if there is no cognitive impairment. Currently, we do not know what impact the ketogenic diet has during various stages, from mild cognitive impairment (MCI) to Alzheimer's disease, but I think it makes more sense for people with symptomatic dementia, not as protection against it. Until then, I prefer the Mediterranean and WFPB diets that have overall health and brain benefits.

The logic of a ketogenic diet comes from the premise that AD might be type 3 diabetes with insulin resistance occurring exclusively in the brain, and by adhering to a ketogenic diet there might be improvement in brain metabolic function because the energy source for nutrition would not rely on insulin.

Ketogenic diets have been around for decades. They are commonly used in other neurological diseases. In fact, prescribing the ketogenic diet is standard treatment for certain forms of epilepsy. Thus, the ketogenic diet is not new to neurology, just new to AD. But it is quite difficult to adhere to for long periods of time, whereas the Mediterranean and WFPB diets are easier to maintain over time.

Gluten and AD

I realize that many nutritionists and doctors see gluten as a major source of nutritional evil, but there is no scientific proof that avoiding gluten (unless you are allergic or intolerant) has any brain benefits. This bit of advice will save you some money at the supermarket!

KEEPING IT REAL: AVOID PROCESSED, REFINED, AND SUGARY FOODS

There's no doubt that the food choices you make can help reduce your risk of heart disease, diabetes, stroke, migraines, arthritis, and, yes, AD. In the earlier section on diabetes you read how sugary drinks like soda contribute to our risk of obesity, type 2 diabetes, and heart disease. But what if I told you that researchers have found that sugar can also damage your brain, producing an unhealthy nutrition-cognition relationship? One such study conducted by Suzanne Craft, PhD, professor of gerontology and geriatric medicine at Wake Forest School of Medicine, found that people who craved and consumed meals that were high in sugar and high in saturated fat (found in foods like beef and bacon) for as little as one month, performed more poorly on memory tests than those who did not. Exactly why certain foods set the stage for mental troubles is a complicated question that researchers are trying to answer now. Although no one knows exactly how much junk food it takes for damage in the brain to begin, scientists agree that eating these foods, especially over a long period of time, isn't just wreaking havoc on our bodies—it might also be shattering our ability to learn, reason, and forge new memories.

Virtually all processed foods contain added sugars for the simple reason that they enhance the flavor and texture at little cost to the manufacturer. Read the labels on products and you will be surprised how often sugar is added to tomato and other sauces during processing. There are at least sixty-one different types of sugar you might find listed on food labels. Keep a watchful eye out for sucrose and high-fructose corn syrup, as well as barley malt, dextrose, maltose, and rice syrup, to name just a few. Sugar is also hidden in condiments (ketchup, relish), flavored yogurts, salad dressings, barbecue sauces, applesauce, and spice mixes. To make matters worse, natural fats, proteins, and fiber are frequently removed when processing foods, which may lead to overeating by disrupting the brain signal that you are full. Have you ever eaten a whole bag of chips in one sitting? Read the ingredients and you'll know why.[3]

Note: Sugar substitutes are no better for you than the real thing— sorry. The reason is, the brain tricks itself into thinking that it's consuming sugar when it's given sweets, which spikes insulin production. So stay away from the artificial sweeteners.

BRAIN DRAIN

If you've ever devoured a frosted cupcake on an empty stomach, you know the sugar rush will eventually be followed by a sugar crash, where you are suddenly tired, irritable, unable to concentrate, and have general brain fog. The good news is, Dr. Craft says an occasional indulgence will not have lasting effects if you eat an otherwise healthy diet. Unfortunately, this is not the case for the typical American, who eats seventy-nine pounds of added sweeteners every year, along with sixty-three pounds of fat (that's equivalent to nearly a full stick of butter every day). With those eating habits, it's no surprise that Americans are suffering from a brain drain. "Negative changes in brain chemistry can occur after just a few weeks of unhealthy eating," Craft says. One of the most toxic effects of chronically consuming foods high in sugar and fat may be the suppression of a brain peptide called BDNF (brain-derived neurotropic factor), which impacts memory and learning. It can create a cascade of chemical reactions that promotes inflammation in the brain, which can damage cells and disrupt connections between neurons.

Even more troubling is the discovery that a diet high in simple sugars, refined carbohydrates, and saturated fats may cause permanent damage by messing with insulin in the brain. Just as in type 2 diabetes, a diet high in saturated fat and sugar can cause brain cells to become insulin resistant, hindering our ability to think and recall, and eventually causing permanent neural damage and possibly AD.[4]

FATS: GOOD, BAD, UNHEALTHY

Just like carbs and cholesterol, there are good fats and there are bad ones. Good fats are those that have not been hydrogenated (the unhealthy process that turns vegetable oils into margarine) and are either monounsaturated or polyunsaturated. They are necessary for proper brain function (it is the major fat in the brain), provide important nutrition, and strengthen our cell walls. Bad fats provide no nutrition whatsoever for the body and can also cause the immune system to malfunction.

Good Fats

Polyunsaturated and monounsaturated are considered good fats. Polyunsaturated fat is found in plant and animal foods, such as salmon, vegetable oils, and some nuts and seeds. Eating moderate amounts of polyunsaturated and monounsaturated fats in place of saturated and trans fats can benefit your brain health.

Examples of healthy fats include:

- Avocado
- Almonds
- Cashews
- Hazelnuts
- Macadamias
- Olive oil

- Peanuts
- Pecans
- Pistachios

Sources of healthy polyunsaturated oils include:

- Omega-3 fatty acids
- Cold-water fish oils (mackerel, salmon, albacore, tuna, sardines, lake trout)
- Flaxseed
- Flaxseed oil
- Pumpkin seeds
- Walnuts

Bad Fats

Examples of bad fats include:

- Partially hydrogenated vegetable oils
- Processed vegetable oils (e.g., soy, canola, corn, cottonseed)
- Saturated fats (e.g. red meat, butter, lard)
- Trans fats (should be avoided completely)

BRAIN-HEALTHY FRUITS AND VEGETABLES

Your mother was right when she told you to eat your fruits and vegetables. Not only are they good for your general health, but researchers in the Chicago Health and Aging Project found a link between vegetable consumption and a lower four-year risk of Alzheimer's. Participants who consumed three servings of vegetables per day had a significantly lower risk of developing the disease than those who consumed less than one serving per day.[5] A serving consists of between a half cup and a full cup, which I know can seem like a lot to many people.

The study showed all types of vegetable consumption is associated with a far slower rate of cognitive decline, but some is particularly beneficial, including sweet potatoes, zucchini, summer squash, eggplant, broccoli, lettuce, celery, apples, and—with the most dramatic impact of all—leafy greens like kale and collards. The Chicago Health and Aging Project concluded that consuming two to four servings of leafy green, yellow, or cruciferous vegetables every day helped protect participants against age-related cognitive decline.

Vegetables and fruits that are dark in color are the best bet for maintaining your cognitive health. ("Cruciferous" are considered among the healthiest veggies you can eat.) In a thirty-year, longitudinal, population-based study published in the *Annals of Neurology*, women who ate the most cruciferous and leafy greens showed a slower rate of cognitive decline than those who ate few or no veggies at all. The following list, which was compiled by the Alzheimer's Association, has been shown to boost cognitive health, so eat up!

Examples of brain-healthy fruits and vegetables include:

Cruciferous	Non-Cruciferous	Fruits
Arugula	Bell peppers	Blueberries
Broccoli	Corn	Blackberries
Brussel's sprouts	Eggplant	Cherries
Bok choy	Onions	Red grapes
Cabbage	Spinach	Oranges
Cauliflower		Plums
Collard greens		Prunes
Kale		Raspberries
Turnips		Strawberries

Protective Properties of Blueberries

If you weren't a big fan of blueberries previously, you might consider becoming one now. In a study published in a 2003 issue of *Nutritional Neuroscience*, blueberry-fed mice that were genetically engineered to develop Alzheimer's disease performed well in mazes and had no changes in amyloid build-up. Researchers concluded that the brain-benefits of blueberries included enhanced memory and neuronal signaling. Other studies found that the polyphenol flavonoids in blueberries, including wild blueberry juice, are able to cross the blood/brain barrier and localize in various brain regions important for learning and memory.

B Vitamins for Brain Health

B vitamins are known as anti-stress vitamins because they help regulate our energy, sleep cycles, and metabolism. They are also needed to create neurotransmitters. Because these vitamins are not stored in our bodies for long, they can become easily depleted, so vitamin B deficiency is common. First, I'll explain what you need to know about B vitamins, then the best way to consume them.

- *Thiamine (B1).* Vitamin B1, which is also referred to as thiamine, is a coenzyme used by the body to metabolize food for energy and to maintain proper heart and nerve function.
- *Pyridoxine (B6).* Vitamin B6 impacts brain function by controlling homocysteine levels, which are not only a risk factor in heart disease but can also damage the neurons in the central nervous system. Vitamin B6 also plays an important role in making the hormones serotonin and norepinephrine, two so-called "happy hormones" that help control our mood, energy, and concentration.

- *Folic Acid (B9).* B9 can help promote healing in the brain by promoting nerve cell regeneration.
- *Cyanocobalamin (B12).* This could be the single most important vitamin for brain health because it allows electrical impulses to transmit quickly and efficiently along the nerve cells. Vitamin B12 benefits our mood, energy level, memory, heart, skin, hair, digestion, and more. It's also an essential vitamin with multiple metabolic functions—including enzyme production, DNA synthesis, hormonal balance, and maintaining a healthy nervous and cardiovascular systems.

The following foods are rich in vitamin B1:[6]

- Asparagus
- Black beans
- Brussels sprouts
- Eggplant
- Green beans
- Green peas
- Lentils
- Lima beans
- Mushrooms
- Oatmeal
- Pinto beans
- Spinach
- Romaine lettuce
- Sunflower seeds
- Tuna
- Tomatoes

These foods are rich in B6:[7]

- Bananas
- Certain fish
- Chicken
- Salmon
- Dried herbs and spices
- Hazelnuts
- Pistachios
- Potatoes
- Raw garlic
- Rice and wheat bran
- Sunflower and sesame seeds
- Spinach
- Turkey
- Vegetable juice

The following foods are rich in B9 (Folic Acid):[8]

- All fortified grains and cereals
- Asparagus
- Broccoli
- Cauliflower
- Leafy greens, like spinach and kale
- Legumes, like lentils, peas, and beans

And these food are rich in B12:[9]

- Beef, lamb, and eggs
- Fatty fish (including caviar)
- Liver (including pâté and sausage)
- Shellfish such as clams, oysters, and mussels have the high
  content; crab and lobster are also a good source.

ANTIOXIDANTS AND AD

Research shows the potential brain-boosting benefits of certain antioxidants, particularly vitamins C and E. As always, it is better to incorporate these nutrients through foods in your diet rather than by supplements, which are not regulated by the FDA. There is no such thing as overdosing on antioxidants in food.

On the contrary, by choosing the right foods, you can lower your "oxidative stress"—an imbalance between the production of free radicals and the ability of the body to detoxify their harmful effects with neutralizing antioxidants. And at the same time, you might possibly reduce your risk of developing Alzheimer's.

SPICE UP YOUR LIFE!

Turmeric

Data suggests that people who live in India have less Alzheimer's per capita when you adjust for age, compared with those who live in the West. Some believe this is due to a low BMI or that many Indians are vegetarian, so they do not consume red meat. Indians also eat large amounts of a spice called turmeric. Turmeric has been used as an ayurvedic treatment for thousands of years to treat colds because it is a ntioxidant and anti-inflammatory. Although studies have yet to prove the health benefits of this spice, it is difficult to argue ears of success!

dicine (also known as Ayurveda) is one of the It originated in India and has evolved United States, Ayurvedic medicine is alth approach.[10]

Cinnamon

Perhaps the most exciting recent dietary finding comes from a new study that reveals that cinnamon has direct anti-Alzheimer's properties, with an ability not only to inhibit the accumulation of the beta-amyloid plaque that leads to Alzheimer's disease but to disassemble plaque that has already formed. That means cinnamon might have both preventive and restorative properties. Cinnamon also alleviates factors associated with Alzheimer's disease by blocking and reversing tau formation in cell cultures.

Other benefits of cinnamon include helping us regulate our metabolism and keeping our insulin levels in check. This delicious spice is being considered as a potential treatment for strokes because of its ability to inhibit cell swelling. Laboratory studies also show that components of cinnamon control production of blood vessels that increase as cancer cells multiply and spread. Human studies involving control subjects and subjects with metabolic syndrome, type 2 diabetes, and polycystic ovary syndrome, all show the healing effects of whole cinnamon. In the form of a bark extract, it can also inhibit viruses such as influenza, herpes, and HIV.[11]

Note: not all studies have shown positive effects of cinnamon, though of course many different variables come into play, including the type and amount of cinnamon and the other drugs subjects are taking.

A Brain Bang for Your Starbucks

Americans love their coffee, so if you are a joe guzzler like me, you'll be pleased to learn that studies have found it to have protective properties against AD. In the Canadian Study of Health and Aging (CSHA), daily coffee drinking lowered Alzheimer's risk by 31 percent during a five-year follow-up. Likewise, the Finland, Italy and the Netherlands Elderly (FINE) study found drinking more than three cups of coffee a day was associated with the least ten-year cognitive decline among elderly men. Additionally, other recent studies have shown that moderate coffee consumption—of dark roast rather than light roast beans—is associated with a reduced risk of type 2 diabetes as well as Alzheimer's disease.

In fact, women with higher coffee consumption over a four-year period experienced less cognitive decline than those consuming little or no coffee. And one of the most convincing of the epidemiologic studies showed that Alzheimer's patients consumed markedly less caffeine (based on dietary reporting) during the twenty years preceding diagnosis, compared with age-matched individuals without Alzheimer's.

Green Tea Gets the Green Light

Green tea is a major source of dietary flavonoids, an antioxidant that seems to be extremely effective at scavenging destructive free radicals, a potential treatment for neurodegenerative disorders. Plus, green tea, like coffee, is high in caffeine and exerts protective effects beyond its antioxidant properties. A recent Japanese study with more than a thousand elderly (seventy-plus years) participants asked them to complete a questionnaire about the frequency of their green tea consumption, which is popular in Japan. The same participants underwent a commonly used memory test. Researchers found that the more green tea the subjects consumed, the lower their rate of cognitive decline. The ones who drank two cups of green tea a day had dramatically lower rates of cognitive impairment than those who only drank three cups a week.

The Good (and Not-So-Great) News About Red Wine

First, the good news for all you oenophiles (wine lovers) out there. Resveratrol, which is found in red wine, has been shown to have anticancer, antiviral, antiaging, anti-inflammatory, and neuroprotective effects.

It has also been reported to be effective against neuronal dysfunction and cell death. When applied to Alzheimer's disease, a recent study in the *Journal of Biological Chemistry* suggests that resveratrol markedly lowers the levels of secreted amyloid peptide produced in different cells. While resveratrol did not stop the production of amyloid, it did promote the degradation of the existing amyloid by breaking down other proteins.[12] Because amyloid protection and plaque formation occurs years before people manifest Alzheimer's symptoms, long-term preventive intake of resveratrol might help with the clearance of the amyloid peptide before plaque is developed and thus delay the onset of AD.

Here's the catch, however. Prevailing wisdom among neurologists now suggests that one needs to drink an enormous amount of red wine in order to get the brain benefits. Red wine contains, at most, 12.59 mg resveratrol per liter, which means you'd need to drink almost forty liters of wine daily. (Meaning your brain might be able to better process the fact that you're too sloshed to stand up at that point!)[13]

Even a 40 mg daily dose of resveratrol, which showed some benefits in a 2010 study published by *Journal of Clinical Endocrinology and Metabolism*, would still require drinking a little over three liters of wine to get sufficient amounts of resveratrol. That's a lot of hooch! Bottom line: a little red wine is good for the soul but not necessarily the best brain booster. And drinking alcohol does not apply to alcoholics, addicts (in recovery or otherwise), or for those who are taking medications for which alcohol is contraindicated (it can produce a fatal cocktail).[14]

CHAPTER 12

Protecting Yourself
Against AD, Part Two:
Physical Activity

MARWAN SABBAGH, MD

It's good for your heart; it's good for your blood pressure; it's good for your waistline. Now, add brain health to the long list of benefits accrued by regular physical activity.

In addition to eating a healthy diet, which is essential in the fight against AD and dementia, scientific evidence clearly shows that vigorous and sustained physical exercise has direct benefits to the brain. In fact, the American Academy of Neurology recommends exercise over medication in the treatment of mild cognitive impairment.[1] For starters, physical activity improves neurochemistry, stimulates brain growth, and even reduces brain shrinkage. In a National Institute of Health–funded study, Jeffrey Burns, MD, of the University of Kansas Alzheimer and

Memory Program, found higher levels of physical exercise is associated with less brain atrophy in people with Alzheimer's disease.

In general, exercise is good for the aging brain. Other studies have shown a positive connection between physical exercise in older adults, including maintenance or enhancement of cognition, especially executive function as well as lower rates of dementia.

When we move our body and our blood starts pumping, our brain is reaping the benefits of rejuvenating blood flow. And while any exercise is better than none, try for two-thirds cardio, one-third strength, depending on your body type. That might translate into a brisk thirty-minute walk four days a week and two resistance-training sessions per week. The increased blood flow physically alters the brain by bathing it in a cascade of growth factors that promote the birth of new brain cells and creates strong neural connections.

Need more proof that what's good for the heart is also good for the brain? Researchers at the University of Gothenburg, Sweden, report that women who scored high on a fitness test in midlife were nearly 90 percent less likely than their moderately fit or unfit peers to develop dementia decades later. Also, the most-athletic women held dementia at bay ten years longer. The study, which appeared in a 2018 issue of *Neurology*, tracked 1,462 women starting in 1968 for more than forty-four years. Each person was given neuropsychological exams and interviews, on average, for twenty-nine years. Women who failed to complete the test ran the highest risk of developing dementia, with 45 percent showing signs of dementia during the follow-up period.[2] The results of this study are consistent with our understanding that poor cardiovascular health may be a factor in our brain health over time. Keep in mind that physical fitness is just one part of the brain health equation and that other lifestyle factors, including diet, also come into play.

HOW MUCH EXERCISE IS ENOUGH?

I realize, as the Bruce Springsteen song says, not everyone is born to run, but hopefully the facts will (literally) change your mind about moving. The recommended amount of heart-pumping (cardio) exercise for healthy adults is thirty minutes a day at least five days a week, according to the American Heart Association guidelines, which the Alzheimer's community has adopted as the model.

The World Health Organization recommends older people do 150 minutes a week of moderate exercise such as brisk walking; seventy-five minutes a week of vigorous aerobic training, like running or dancing; or a combination of the two. If time (or lack of enthusiasm) is an issue, you can break up your thirty-minute-a-day regimen by doing ten minutes of aerobic exercise three times daily, perhaps in the morning, afternoon, and evening. Try not to increase your heart rate too close to your bedtime because it might make it more difficult to sleep. In general, however, adding exercise to our day helps us sleep better, working like a natural sleep aid.

Of course, you should check with your doctor before starting any exercise program to determine what is safe, depending on your or your family member's condition, especially if Alzheimer's has been diagnosed. Your doctor can help you create a plan that's right for you.

STAYING ACTIVE IMPROVES
QUALITY OF LIFE

In addition to the brain benefits of exercise, new research suggests that working up a good sweat may even improve the quality of life for people with Alzheimer's. The effects were modest, but a series of studies found vigorous workouts by people with mild memory impairment decreased the levels of a warped protein linked to the risk of getting Alzheimer's for people who were still in early stages of the disease.

"Regular aerobic exercise could be a fountain of youth for the brain," said cognitive neuroscientist Laura Baker, PhD, of Wake Forest School of Medicine, at the 2015 Alzheimer's Association International Conference. Baker studied seventy-one previously sedentary older adults who showed symptoms of the mild cognitive impairment (MCI) that is known to increase the risk of developing Alzheimer's. They were given monitors to wear while doing cardio exercises to ensure that they got their heart rate up, and a control group kept their heart rate deliberately low while doing simple stretch classes. MRI scans showed the exercisers experienced increased blood flow in brain regions important for memory and thought processing, while cognitive tests showed improvement in their attention, planning, and organizing abilities and other so-called executive functions. Equally encouraging were tests of the participants' spinal fluid that also showed reduced levels of tau protein in exercisers over age seventy.[3]

COGNITIVE TRAINING: CHANGING IT UP

In addition to keeping your body fit, it is important to keep your mind in shape by being your own personal cognitive trainer. According to the National Academy of Sciences, the term *cognitive training* is used to indicate a broad set of interventions, including those aimed at enhancing reasoning (such as problem solving), memory, and speed of processing (for example, speed of identifying visual information on a screen). Such structured training exercises may or may not be computer based. Some evidence, based largely on a single, long-duration clinical trial, indicated that cognitive training can improve long-term cognitive function and help maintain independence, including daily living activities.

The data is robust that cognitive stimulation has brain benefits, but this might not include what you think. While tests suggest that those people engaging in brain teasers, such as sudoku or crossword puzzles, do better cognitively than those who did not, the problem with these kinds of brain games is that the benefits are temporary, limited to a specific activity, and can be socially isolating. If you do only one activity, say crosswords for example, you'll get very good at the puzzles, but your learning curve will flatten along with the mental benefits. While mental stimulation, whether it's online tests for attention or sudoku, is certainly better than staring passively at the TV or scrolling through Facebook on your phone, the repetition of that activity will strengthen only one neural pathway, not others. Plus, we don't know how long the brain benefits last once you stop or log off. There's no proof, for example, that doing two hours of crosswords versus one hour will be twice as protective against dementia. Similarly, there is no evidence to support the notion that these kinds of beneficial long-term cognitive effects are obtained with commercial, computer-based "brain-training" applications, which appear to have short-term benefits that apply only to the specific cognitive task that is rehearsed.

The trick to staying mentally sharp is to mix it up. Trying new things is what makes more neural connections. One of the best ways to activate your brain is to challenge it with something you've never done before. Learning new skills—such as speaking a different language, whipping up an original recipe, learning to play an instrument, digging into a new book, dancing (a double benefit because you're remembering steps and moving), traveling somewhere you've never been before, woodworking, or singing in a choir—will give you a feeling of satisfaction and accomplishment that you can't get from a video game. You're expanding your horizons (and neural pathways) and developing life skills that will enhance your mental agility and, perhaps, your quality of life.

BE MINDFUL WITH MEDITATION

Meditation is increasingly popular these days. It is a form of cognitive training because you are teaching the brain how to relax and let go. Much has been reported about the mind-body connection, including studies that have clearly shown meditation can help reduce stress in as little as twenty minutes a day. I know that I said exercise is good for your brain, but there are also a whole lot of mental benefits in just sitting still and breathing. Long-time meditators have shown improved brain function that comes from firing up the neurons, and this increased activity in the prefrontal cortex is associated with positive emotions. There are numerous traditions and no right way to meditate, so you should find a practice that works for you and stick with it. According to one meditation teacher, Light Watkins, author of *Bliss More: How to Succeed in Meditation Without Really Trying*, you don't have to sit soldier-straight, Buddha-style with total darkness and silence in order to get the full meditative benefits. He suggests supporting your back with a pillow, on your bed, in a chair, or wherever you feel comfortable, and breathe normally with your eyes closed. It's okay if you fall asleep the first few times, but eventually you'll be able to meditate while keeping your mind awake and alert. Start with five minutes and work your way up to twenty minutes a day. For many, selecting a word, prayer, sound, or mantra that you find soothing and peaceful will help quiet your thoughts. Like exercise, the more you do, the better you'll feel.[4]

"By combining breath regulation, deep relaxation and meditation, we literally shift the balance of our stress regulation systems in our brain and our body," explains Sat Bir Singh Khalsa, PhD, a Harvard neuroscientist and author of *Your Brain on Yoga*. "Meditation affects the activity of our genes, lowers our heart rate and blood pressure, and decreases the production of stress hormones, which results in lower symptoms of mental and physical distress."[5]

And let's not forget, deep prayer (not just a quick blessing over the dinner table) and yoga breathing are also ways to practice this mindfulness training.

SOCIALIZE

While we don't know exactly why, having an active social life is good for the brain as well as for people at risk for AD. Studies have shown that feeling a part of a family, a circle of friends, and a community (workplace, religious, social, or political groups) throughout our lifetime helps stave off depression and, of course, loneliness while keeping our minds vibrant.

Research at the Cleveland Clinic concurs that a rich social network provides sources of support, reduces stress, combats depression, and enhances intellectual stimulation. Studies have shown that those with the most social interaction within their community experience the slowest rate of memory decline. Happy marriages, long-term relationships, and having a purpose in life have shown significant protective effects against age-related cognitive impairment. Here are some more supportive findings:

- Did you know that Britain has a minister of loneliness? Apparently, research found more than nine million people in the country often or always feel lonely, according to a 2017 report published by the Jo Cox Commission on Loneliness.[6] The issue prompted Prime Minister Theresa May to appoint a minister for loneliness. "I want to confront this challenge for our society and for all of us to take action to address the loneliness endured by the elderly, by caregivers, by those who have lost loved ones," she said in a statement.[7] Mark Robinson, the chief officer of Age UK, Britain's largest charity working with older people, warned that the problem could be fatal.[8] "It's proven to be worse for health than smoking 15 cigarettes a day, but it can be overcome and needn't be a factor in older people's lives," Robinson told a reporter for *The New York Times*.[9] Similarly, a former United States surgeon general, Dr. Vivek Murthy, wrote an article for the *Harvard Business Review* in 2017 arguing that loneliness can be associated "with a greater risk of cardiovascular disease, dementia, depression and anxiety."[10] Studies seem to back this up.

- In a 2010 study of 193 Maryland nursing home residents diagnosed with dementia, researcher J. Cohen-Mansfield and colleagues found that those who were given more social interaction with other people (versus nonhuman stimuli) were significantly more attentive and displayed a far more positive attitude.[11]
- The nearly decade-long 2009 Rush Memory and Aging Project found that elderly participants who had the least amount of social contact had a 40 percent increased risk of developing disabilities.
- A three-year study of more than two thousand women aged seventy-eight and older, which appeared in the 2005 issue of the *American Journal of Public Health*, concluded that larger social networks have a protective influence on cognitive function among elderly women.
- According to a study published in the 2009 issue of *Neurology*, middle-aged people who lived isolated lifestyles were more prone to cognitive decline as they age than those who socialized.

So cherish your friends and loved ones, get out and circulate, join a book club (reading is good for the brain), go to a meet-up with people who have similar interests (meetup.com), volunteer for a charity or cause you believe in, talk to people who have different views and backgrounds than you do (remember what I said about mixing it up?), have a regular girls or boys night out, play team sports or tennis, have a regular card game night, or fall in love! It's never too late to bathe your brain in dopamine and endorphins, those neurotransmitters that create that natural high while improving our focus and drive![12]

GET AN ANNUAL BODY CHECKUP
AND ONE FROM THE NECK UP

In addition to following the advice in this book for decreasing your risk of diabetes and stroke, and keeping your weight and BMI in check, one of the ways to catch early symptoms of brain and other health changes is to get a yearly checkup. Most insurance policies pay for an annual checkup by a primary care doctor that includes weight/BMI, blood work, blood pressure, and heart monitoring via electrocardiograms. Bring a list of your medications (including supplements) and be honest and open about your lifestyle. Your doctor is there to help not to judge, so withholding information hurts only you.

When there are any red flags after getting your results back, you will be referred to the appropriate specialists. If you're feeling depressed see a therapist, which as you read, helped Jamie during a dark period. If you are on Medicare, you can get additional coverage by signing up for part B, for which you pay a monthly premium. It covers most medically necessary doctors' services, preventive care, medical equipment, hospital outpatient services, laboratory tests, X-rays, mental-health care, and some home health and ambulance services. Do your research about getting this supplemental insurance for Medicare in your state.

Yearly Wellness Visits

Generally as part of a wellness visit, your provider will ask you to fill out a questionnaire, called a "Health Risk Assessment." Answering these questions can help you and your provider develop a personalized prevention plan to help you stay healthy and get the most out of your visit. It can also include:

- A review of your medical and family history
- Developing or updating a list of current providers and prescriptions
- Height, weight, blood pressure, and other routine measurements
- Detection of any cognitive impairment
- Personalized health advice
- A list of risk factors and treatment options for you
- A screening schedule (like a checklist) for appropriate preventive services. Get details about coverage for screenings, shots, and other preventive services.
- Advance care planning

You pay nothing for the "Welcome to Medicare" preventive visit or the yearly wellness visit if your doctor or other qualified health-care provider accepts your insurance. The part B deductible doesn't apply. You may have to pay coinsurance, and the part B deductible may apply if your doctor or other health-care provider performs additional tests or services during the same visit. These additional tests or services aren't covered under the preventive benefits.[13]

Sense-ible Advice

Very often, eye and hearing exams are easy to overlook on the long list of health and medical to-dos, especially if you or a loved one is dealing with AD.

But sensory deficit—loss of vision and hearing—are common problems among older adults. And they also magnify the appearance of cognitive problems. In other words, not being able to see or hear well makes the cognitive issues seem worse (even though sensory deficit doesn't contribute to AD).

So make sure you or loved ones take protective steps: have a hearing and vision test. Get eyewear, and in the case of hearing aids, which I realize are very expensive, look at other options. There are less expensive alternatives on the market that can help with hearing.

CHAPTER 13

A World Without
Alzheimer's? Yes!

MARWAN SABBAGH, MD

I t was front-page news all over the country, even though you could read the caution, even skepticism, behind the headlines.

"New Alzheimer's Drug Slows Memory Loss in Early Trial Results" was the page one head in *The New York Times*.

"Experimental Alzheimer's drug stirs hope," read the story on CNN .com.

"New Alzheimer's drug shows hints on progress," said *Science* magazine.

This big-deal drug called "BAN2401"—developed by Biogen Inc. in Cambridge, Massachusetts, and Eisai Co., Ltd. in Tokyo—was shown to slow the pace of cognitive decline and reverse the buildup of amyloid, which, as we know, is implicated in the progression of the disease.

I was in the audience when the results of the BAN2401 trial were presented at the 2018 Alzheimer's Association annual conference in

Chicago. I was later quoted in *USA Today* about the announcement. I predicted that the new findings would "energize the field."

As the cautiously optimistic tone of the media reports (and my comment) suggest, the field needed a little spark. The widespread perception is that Alzheimer's research has been one long string of failures, and those of us who investigate treatments for it have been like a baseball team mired in an extended slump.

The truth is, while it's rare to get this kind of mainstream media attention, Alzheimer's research has actually been very productive, particularly in the last decade. If I may be allowed another baseball metaphor, we don't knock many balls out of the park, but we've been hitting a lot of singles and doubles. Over the past ten years or so, we've been chipping away at the puzzle that is AD, and we've been making steady, incremental progress to the point that I can now offer an honest and upbeat answer to the question I get almost every day from patients who come into my office.

"Is there hope?" they ask me. For themselves. For their moms, dads, husbands, and wives.

My answer: absolutely yes.

And I don't mean that in the you-should-never-give-up-hope sense. I'm saying that there's now legitimate reason to be optimistic. Not about curing or preventing Alzheimer's. That also may come in the not-too-distant future, but what I'm talking about is the sea change in the way we are viewing the disease. After decades of study and numerous setbacks, we now have a firmer grasp of how the disease disrupts the brain. That has led to potential Alzheimer's treatments, which in turn means that Alzheimer's patients may now face a course of interventions similar to those with certain types of cancers, rheumatoid arthritis, and HIV/AIDS.

In other words, like those diseases, we may be moving toward a model in which Alzheimer's may not be curable, but it is treatable.

That means that someone diagnosed with AD might soon be able to live a long, symptom-free life, given the right treatment. I've selected some of the latest, most promising trials and studies for this chapter to show you where the field is heading. Keep in mind, there will be many more by the time you read this book.

I realize some of this may be a bit technical, and the names of some of these new drugs may sound as though they were cooked up by a science-fiction writer. But I assure there is nothing fictional here. This is fact—exciting, important fact. As a researcher, I want you to be armed with the best possible information, not only for your own education on AD, but so that you will be better equipped to have a conversation with your physician about some of these options for you or your loved one.

DRUG TESTS TO PREVENT MEMORY LOSS OR ALZHEIMER'S DEMENTIA IN THOSE AT HIGHER RISK

Because Alzheimer's-related brain changes often take place decades before symptoms appear, scientists are trying to intervene at the earliest possible stage in order to stop or slow the progression of the disease. New classes of drugs are being designed to address this key problem. Here's a brief roundup of some of them, as you may hear your doctor mention them.

The A4 Study

The A4 trial is an important clinical trial in several respects. First, it will determine if it can prevent memory loss from progressing into Alzheimer's disease by treating older individuals who may be at a higher risk (because they have amyloid detected on scans) with the drug solane-zumab. This medication was found in earlier studies to help people with mild Alzheimer's dementia, with a 34 percent reduction in the rate of decline, but did not work in people with moderate dementia. It might be more effective when it was given earlier in the course of the disease. Solanezumab has not been approved for AD dementia.[1]

Researchers are testing eleven thousand adults, using a PET scan, for an elevated level of amyloid plaque in their brain. People who do not show evidence of elevated amyloid in their brains will not be able to participate. This group will not receive the IV infusion of solanezumab or a placebo but will complete the same memory tests every six months to compare changes in cognition over time. The drug used in A4 was found to be safe in the most recent studies, but more research needs to be done.

At this writing, the A4 study has completed enrollment and is ongoing. For more information, contact www.a4study.org/about/.

The TOMMORROW Study

This study that began in 2013 had two goals. One was to see if a new genetic test can determine whether subjects were at risk of developing mild cognitive dementia due to Alzheimer's (MCI-AD) within five years. The other goal was to look at the effectiveness of the drug pioglitazone (approved as Actos to treat diabetes) in delaying the onset of MCI-AD in cognitively normal people who are at high risk.

This trial was conducted worldwide and enrolled approximately 3,500 subjects. Participants were assigned to high- or low-risk groups for developing MCI-AD, based on the results of the biomarker risk algorithm. In other words, they were selected for participation on the basis of their genetic risk profile. Volunteers in the high-risk group were randomly assigned to one of the two treatment groups, which were not known to the participant and study doctor during the study (unless there was an urgent medical need). Those in the low-risk group were assigned a placebo. Results of this study are currently being evaluated.[2]

The EARLY Trial

This study used a different type of drug to assess the risk associated with the buildup of amyloid plaques and the latest technological advances to measure the amount of amyloid in the brain. Stopping or slowing down amyloid plaque formation may delay memory loss associated with Alzheimer's disease. It may also help control other changes in the cells of the brain that contribute to the disease. Keep in mind that a buildup of amyloid plaques does not mean that symptoms of Alzheimer's disease will develop in the next few weeks, months, or even years, but the data clearly shows that having amyloid in the brain increases the risk of future progression.

The purpose of the EARLY trial was to evaluate the safety and efficacy of an investigational medication, a BACE inhibitor (more about them in a moment), in people at risk of developing AD. This was an oral medication developed to stop the production of amyloid. It has shown promise in animal models of AD. Recently, the study was suspended because of concerns about liver damage, but other drugs in the class are currently being developed.

DRUG TRIAL FOR EARLY-STAGE ALZHEIMER'S DEMENTIA

In addition to potentially preventive medications, there are many drugs being developed to treat AD in the symptomatic phase of the dementia. So-called "monoclonal drugs" are being tested with an eye toward slowing disease progression. These are synthetic proteins given intravenously and are specifically designed to find, target, and clear amyloid plaques. One such experimental drug currently in clinical trials is crenezumab, which is for people with early to mild Alzheimer's disease. Investigators are assessing the drug's safety and efficacy by evaluating any changes in participants' dementia rating and performance through neuropsychological tests. Crenezumab is an antibody that finds amyloid, binds to it, and removes it from the brain. In studies of mild AD dementia, participants receiving crenezumab clearly showed a slowing in the rate of decline compared to a placebo. This drug is undergoing more extensive clinical trials and, if successful, could be approved within three to five years.

Its cousin gantenerumab, also an antibody, is also being tested in large clinical trials at present. Gantenerumab has two advantages that make it appealing. One, it has been shown to consistently remove amyloid as detected on PET scans (scans that can detect the amyloid directly). Two, it can be given as an injection, similar to a flu shot, meaning there is no need for an IV infusion.

Another hard-to-pronounce but potentially important drug currently being investigated is called aducanumab. One early randomized, double-blind clinical trial enrolled 192 predementia and mild Alzheimer's patients at various sites in the United States. It aimed to assess the safety and effect of the drug at different doses compared to a placebo. The results were measured through PET imaging to determine how much amyloid was cleared and if symptom decline began to stabilize.

Interim results from the first 165 patients have been published in the scientific journal *Nature*. All monthly doses were seen to significantly reduce amyloid plaques in the brain, whereas little to no change was seen in the placebo group after one year. The higher the doses, the greater the reduction of plaque. The drug also appeared to slow the rate of cognitive decline, the first time that a drug showed a correlation between removal of target pathology and stabilization of clinical symptoms. This is a very exciting development!

Results from the long-term extension part of the trial were presented at the 2017 Clinical Trials on Alzheimer's disease (CTAD) meeting. Patients given aducanumab have continued to experience a time-and dose-dependent reduction in amyloid plaque levels.

There are also two large-scale, randomized, double-blind, and placebo-controlled Phase III clinical trials for people with early stage

AD underway. One aims to enroll 1,350 patients at 187 sites in North America, Australia, Europe, and Asia. The other would like to enlist the same number of patients at 194 sites in North America, Europe, and Asia. Both trials will assess the efficacy of aducanumab in treating the symptoms of Alzheimer's disease. These trials are expected to conclude in 2022.

STOPPING THE PRODUCTION OF AMYLOID

Not all promising new medications pan out, or at least not initially.

I mentioned BACE inhibitors earlier. These are a class of drugs that, instead of trying to remove the amyloid already present in the brain, works to stop the production of the protein itself. This is appealing for two reasons:

First, it is an oral medication (a pill) and is not administered via IV or injection.

Second, it targets the production of amyloid before it becomes a plaque or potentially causes damage. And one of the themes you've heard me hit again and again in this book is that the earlier we can intervene in the Alzheimer's disease process the better.

Unfortunately, this class of drugs has, so far, been shown to be ineffective or have toxic effects on the liver. Until more results are in, all anti-amyloid treatments are still inconclusive as researchers continue to study and interpret biomarker data.

Does that mean that all the appealing aspects of the BACE inhibitors can be kissed goodbye? Not at all. It may sound like a cliché, but failure is part of the scientific process. I have full confidence that some of the new drugs and treatments that have not yet panned out may, with modifications and new approaches, turn out to be valuable.

RAGE COMPOUNDS

Despite its name, RAGE is an exciting, new potential AD treatment that has nothing to do with anger issues. It stands for "receptor for advanced glycation end" products. What does this mean? In part, it has to do with oxidative stress and free radicals that can cause our cells and tissues to stop functioning properly and have serious consequences for our brain and our health. RAGE has been shown in people with diabetes and could be one of the ties between AD and dementia. In fact, RAGE compounds are also being explored for the treatment of AD.

Two RAGE medications are being investigated but are in different stages of development. Low doses of the drug azeliragon have shown promising benefits, including slowing cognitive decline in preliminary studies. There has been some conflicting data, however, which showed a failure rate in some subjects, while others did significantly better on the drug compared to subjects treated with a placebo. Scientists are hotly debating the benefits of RAGE, and additional studies so far have failed to reproduce exciting evidence of benefit.

TARGET THE TAU

For more than a decade, many researchers have believed tau—not amyloid—is the real driver of AD symptoms and progression such as memory loss and dementia, or at least an important accomplice, since tau levels correlate with clinical progression better than amyloid. Although the amyloid-tau debate still continues among scientists in the AD field, new tau-targeting treatments are being done that can lead to better diagnostic tools. Anti-tau immunotherapy is an area where numerous clinical trials are being conducted. Preliminary results have demonstrated great promise for their use, which I have studied extensively. There are two current vaccines undergoing investigation that have been found to be both safe and effective in preclinical trials. The ability to trigger an immune response that can target hazardous tau has the potential to provide both therapeutic and preventive benefits. The future of immunotherapy includes developing vaccines like these that target the formation of pathologic tau. Data from current clinical trials will shed light on safety, tolerability, and efficacy in humans.

Microtubule (an important part of the cellular process) stabilizers are another class of drugs directed toward tau. This class of drugs has demonstrated the greatest potential with the ability to target tau protein that may prevent AD dementia symptoms as well as help patients with MCI. Research includes evaluating the gross density of neurofibrillary tangles, improvements in cognitive and behavioral testing, and the total tau and composite tau levels.

Methylene blue, which sounds like something out of the TV series *Breaking Bad*, has been used in the past to treat cyanide poisoning. In its current investigative formulation LMTX, it is the most advanced clinical trial for tau treatments to date, but results so far are mixed and not consistently positive. The premise revolves around inhibition of tau clusters. The ability of these drugs to be tolerated along with inhibiting pathologic tau aggregation can provide a broad approach to tau therapy. Further research on this class of drug is ongoing.

PERSONALIZED COGNITIVE THERAPY

Another exciting new development in the fight against AD is what's called personalized cognitive rehabilitation therapy, or CogStim, which can help people with early-stage dementia significantly maintain their ability to engage in daily activities. Cognitive rehabilitation involves a therapist working with people who have dementia and a family caregiver to identify issues where they would like to see improvements. Together they set up to three goals, and then the therapist helps develop strategies to achieve these goals. A large-scale University of Exeter, England, study presented at the Alzheimer's Association International Conference in 2017 found cognitive rehabilitation helps people with dementia improve and maintain their normal functioning and independence.

The goals participants chose were varied, as dementia affects people in different ways. Some subjects wanted to find ways of staying independent by learning or relearning how to use household appliances or cellphones. Some wanted to manage simple everyday tasks better. Others wanted to stay socially connected and focused on being able to remember the names of friends or relatives, or to improve their ability to engage in conversation. Several strategies targeted safety issues, such as remembering to lock the door or how to withdraw money at a cash machine.

The researchers found that those who took part in the therapy showed significant improvement in the areas they had identified after both the ten-week and follow-up sessions. Both participants and caregivers were happy with the subjects' improvements in the areas they identified. Dr. Ola Kudlicka, who managed the trial, told a reporter from the *Science Daily*, "Contrary to popular belief, our trial shows that people with early-stage dementia, given the right kind of support, have the capacity to learn and to improve their skills." The Alzheimer's Society is funding an implementation study so the researchers can work with social-care providers to adapt the therapy for use in nursing home and memory facilities. The personalized nature of this therapy shows that tailoring approaches to care and setting individual goals can be beneficial to both patient and caregiver.[3]

FINAL THOUGHTS

As you can see from our overview of the latest AD research, there are many promising new drugs and therapies emerging. We can now identify people like Jamie who are at risk, thanks to the emergence of genetic science. We may now be able to talk about treating Alzheimer's with disease-modifying drugs, of which we hope BAN2401 may be the first.

Thanks to the efforts of many, from major organizations like the Alzheimer's Association to individual advocates like Jamie, we are now seeing the kind of interest, support, and funding that is critical to scientific progress. The announcement in July 2018 that a group of philanthropists, including Bill Gates, have created a thirty million dollar accelerate fund to support the development of new Alzheimer's diagnostics is another important and welcome step in that direction.

These are all huge developments in the field. But let's not stop there. I think we can now begin to strategize about a future without Alzheimer's disease.

We know the changes occur decades before the onset of symptoms. Researchers like me speculate that interceding before an individual becomes symptomatic would be the optimal approach. We are trying to prove that early intervention will work. How early and what forms would that take? Let me paint you a scenario.

Imagine a day when we can take a drop of blood or a cheek swab from an infant and look at DNA to identify the risk of getting Alzheimer's disease many years later.

Imagine in young and middle adulthood, we can vaccinate against the development of Alzheimer's, as we now do for mumps and polio.

Imagine in late adulthood we can prescribe medications that prevent the onset of the disease altogether.

We would save millions of lives and trillions of dollars.

If you think this is purely wishful thinking, you should know that everything I have just mentioned is being investigated. It might take years or even decades before this becomes a reality, but we are working on it. At the moment, we are losing millions of people to Alzheimer's, and we spend a huge amount of money (as well as blood, sweat, and tears) caring for them.

As I've said, we are now entering a period when newly diagnosed Alzheimer's patients may have a wide array of options for effectively treating and managing the disease. But look a little farther down the road, and I can easily envision a future in which there are no more memory-care assisted-living facilities because there are no more dementia sufferers to inhabit them. This is the goal.

In the meantime, the message here is hope and nonpassive engagement, hope that we will soon make massive medical progress that might one day end Alzheimer's or at least make a significant reduction or delay in the disease. Active engagement is essential as a tool of empowerment. We know there is growing evidence that we can modify risk by making certain lifestyle changes, as seen in the large studies included in this book. Our challenge is trying to prove that these strategies to delay AD work at the individual level and to raise the funds and harness the enthusiasm, hard work, and sacrifice to make this dream a reality.

In life, we don't get to pick our parents or our gene pool. But we are coming to an era that we can alter the footprint and impact of our genetic makeup. This growing field of research is called "epigenetics." It is a field of study where scientists determine how the environment (stress, sleep, food, exercise, medications, and so forth) impacts genes. We cannot manipulate genes yet, but someday we might be able to turn off genes associated with AD risk altogether. If we win that fight, we would be living in a world where Alzheimer's disease would be a rarely seen plague of the past, as unfamiliar to a future society as smallpox or polio is to ours.

Yes, a world without Alzheimer's disease. A world without millions living in the shadows. Wouldn't that be a slice of heaven on earth?

CHAPTER 14

Hear Me Roar

t's 7:30 a.m., July 19, 2018, in room 101 at MRI Services, University of California–San Diego Radiology Services.

"Where are my glasses?" my mom says as she examines the various release forms she's been asked to read and sign.

"Mom," I reply. "They're on your head."

She smiles sheepishly. "That's the worst place I could have put them!"

Flipping down her glasses over her eyes, she finishes the paperwork. Soon she's summoned into the interior of the office for her MRI. Step one in a long day—actually a long week—in which, at her own request, Mom would undergo cognitive testing at the university that, through my volunteer work with Mary Sundsmo at the Alzheimer's Disease Research Center (ADRC), has been such an important part of my life in recent years.

On this misty morning, I've driven her from my house in Ramona down to San Diego to begin the process. My eyes were a bit misty too. Would this be yet another close and beloved relative—my mom, for heaven's sakes—afflicted by Alzheimer's? Please say no.

It has been forty-eight years since our memorable family road trip to

177

visit her relatives in Iowa—a lifetime ago. I've never forgotten the stories Mom told us about her childhood and her time with Great-Grandma Neva, as we rolled through the American West in the family Ford station wagon.

Nor had I forgotten the nursing home horror of coming face-to-face with Neva and, for the first time, with a disease that would later haunt my life.

My mom, of course, is aware of the events that have transpired in my life since 2009, the events that constitute this book. But now it is she who needs my help.

Now seventy-eight, Mom lives alone in the town of Chico in Northern California. After splitting up with my father, she had married her high school sweetheart, Vincent Zemis. A former professional baseball player, he was also a good and caring man, and when he died in 2014, I felt my mom going into a bit of a tailspin. I noticed that she, though highly intelligent, would start to mix up dates, facts, and names. Losing the glasses on her head was a small example. I was concerned. I'd already watched one parent slip into the grasp of Alzheimer's. I couldn't bear the thought of the same thing happening to my mom.

Her MRI complete, we headed over to her appointment with Dr. James Brewer, who is the chairman of the Department of Neurosciences at UCSD's School of Medicine. A highly distinguished researcher and a colleague and friend of my coauthor Dr. Marwan Sabbagh, Dr. Brewer is also a gentle and genial presence whom I suspect has made difficult exams a little easier for many anxious patients and families, no matter what the results.

He began asking my mom questions, as if it were polite, casual conversation between two people meeting at a dinner party, not a distinguished neurologist probing to see whether a patient was showing signs of a debilitating illness.

"What did you do for a living, Suzanne?" he asked Mom.

She replied that after her divorce from my dad, she had gone to work at West Coast University in Irvine, a private college focused on health care.

"Interesting. What did you do there?"

Mom grinned. "I was Miss-cellaneous. I did everything."

Dr. Brewer chuckled. "Ah, puns are intact. Very good!"

Mom then proceeded, with résumé-like precision, to rattle off the various positions, years, and institutions she had worked in during her years in higher education. She had started as a receptionist at West Coast, eventually became associate registrar, and concluded her career years later as assistant director of Alumni Relations at Loyola University Law School in Los Angeles.

"I retired in 2004," she concluded.

"Very good," said Dr. Brewer. "So do you now live alone?"

"Does my puppy count?"

Again, Dr. Brewer chuckled. Mom told him about her granddaughter (my niece) who has three children and lives nearby in Chico.

"Ah," said Dr. Brewer, "so you're a great-grandmother!"

"I am," Mom said proudly. "I have three great-grandchildren: two boys, twelve and fourteen, and a girl who just turned four."

Dr. Brewer put down his notebook and smiled admiringly, looking at me and Mom. "That's good," he said, "a really detailed story of your life."

I beamed like a proud parent—funny how the roles reverse as we get older—but Mom was still concerned. She's always been a big reader and talked to Dr. Brewer about some of her issues. "When there are more than two characters in a novel, I lose track," she said. "And sometimes I'm reading words incorrectly." She cites a specific example of a magazine article she had read about a famous mountaineer. "I read the word *avalanche* as *advanced*," she said. "That really bothered me!"

"Has your vision changed?" Dr. Brewer asked.

"Not at all. Also, I've lost the ability to do math in my head. I can still balance my checkbook, but it's become more difficult."

"How long has that gone on?"

"About a year."

Now it was my turn to chime in, as Mom has consented to have me present. "I've noticed she'll sometimes tell me the same story."

"Not within five minutes or so?" Dr. Brewer asked.

"No, usually within twenty-four hours."

He didn't seem too concerned with that or with Mom leaving her glasses on her head on the morning of a medical procedure. In fact, he seemed quite pleased with all her responses. "I have to tell you," he said. "I don't see any red flags. There's really nothing happening here, except—"

"Except that I'm getting old," Mom interrupted, finishing his sentence.

Dr. Brewer grinned, then pulled up the results of the MRI on a screen in the exam room. He pointed to the two small lobes on either side. "This is the hippocampus," he said. "It's critical to the construction of memory. It's one of the first things ravaged by Alzheimer's disease."

I was aware of that, but I saw Mom leaning forward, eager to learn.

"For a seventy-eight-year-old," he said, pointing to the lobes. "That's a beautiful-looking hippocampus."

"Well, that's great . . . I guess."

"Mom," I joked, "you can bring these with you and use them as a pickup line in Starbucks. 'Hey, handsome, want to see my hippocampus?'"

She rolled her eyes.

"Seriously," I said, addressing Dr. Brewer, "what do you think?"

Based on the interview and the MRI, he said, "I wouldn't say it completely rules out AD, but it's good evidence."

There is still much more testing to go. Mom's balance and coordination will be gauged; she'll undergo a complete physical, and there will be more in-depth psychological and cognitive evaluation.

As for her forgetfulness, Dr. Brewer discovered one possible culprit when he looked over a list of my mom's medications. After back surgery a few years ago, she was prescribed an antidepressant, amitriptyline, to help her sleep. This, he told us, has been shown to interfere with neurotransmitters in the brain. "While it may have been appropriate medication in the weeks following the surgery, I'm not sure you still need to be on that," Dr. Brewer said in his understated style.

He also thought my mom could use some physical therapy to help with her balance. Later we would find out that Mom had some mild cognitive impairment (MCI) due to vascular issues. Her years of smoking might have contributed to this. Fortunately, it's treatable, and just another example of why early diagnosis is important!

I listened to what Dr. Brewer said that day and nodded. My mom is indeed aging, and like most people approaching eighty, she has some health issues. Despite that, I'm doing internal cartwheels of joy. I'm thankful because, unlike her grandmother, unlike her mother, and unlike her first husband, my mom does not have Alzheimer's disease.

But what about me?

In a few years, I will soon be approaching the likely onset age for those with my genetic 4/4 profile. So do I freak out sometimes when I misplace my keys or forget a name? You betcha. But the difference now is that I don't let it ruin my day or rule my life.

I find my keys, the name comes to me eventually, and I chalk it up to normal aging and move on.

I'm very positive about my future and with some good reasons. B.A.B.E.S. is going strong. We are now sponsoring a support group at the ADRC for those who learn their genetic status. I sit in on this group and hear stories similar to mine. The people in the group come to us bewildered, uncertain, often terrified. The first step is to validate those feelings, which we do. Then we talk about research opportunities, about lifestyle, about, well, doing a lot of the same things I've done over the past decade. I hope our program will inspire similar support groups around the country.

Speaking of lifestyle, as you've read in Marwan's chapter on protecting ourselves from AD, the evidence is more and more compelling about the benefits of a healthy diet, physical activity, and so forth. I admit I'm not perfect in that area, but I make a conscious effort to eat healthy, and as of this writing, I'm getting back to the gym and the yoga classes that I so enjoy.

My advocacy work continues to keep me busy. I'm currently on a working group of the combined National Institute on Aging and National Institutes of Health (NIH/NIA) that is looking at the thorny issue of genetic and biomarker disclosure. Our task is to develop recommendations on how and when such information should be disclosed.

I'm also still involved with UsAgainstAlzheimer's and their network WomenAgainstAlzheimer's, and we're still making our voices heard in Washington where, I am happy to say, people are now listening. Every year since our initial summit in 2013, the amount of government funding for AD research has increased. It's going to those scientists studying the kind of promising treatments that Marwan detailed in the previous chapter, which is further cause for optimism. And I still continue to speak to national audiences, including the National Association of Genetic Counselors and the Medical School of Miami, to name a couple.

Yet, despite my continued work in the Alzheimer's arena, I'm trying hard to find a balance in my life. While I'm committed to the cause, it doesn't mean I necessarily need to be thinking about plaques and tangles, studies and funding every waking hour, as it sometimes seems. Recently, Doug and I decided to downsize. Like many couples our age, we're going to sell our house and find a smaller place. As much as I love Ramona and will continue to visit this wonderful community, I suspect we may end up going down the hill and finding a small place near the water in San Diego. Being on a boat is meditative for me, so I rationalize that it's probably good for my brain health to include a boat as part of my plan.

But the truth is, as much I stand ready to support and help those who are battling AD, part of the way I'm learning to deal with the specter of the disease is by not obsessing about it. Or at least not as much as I did a few years back.

Lead a balanced life. That's what we're trying to do—and that's what I tell others fighting AD. Here are some of the other things I've learned during my Alzheimer's odyssey. May they guide you along yours.

OPEN YOUR HEART TO THE KINDNESS OF OTHERS

During the period when I was in a downward spiral after the devastating news of my 4/4 genetic status, I found support, warmth, and kindness from many people. Similarly, when my family and I were struggling with my dad's AD, I was touched by the responses from strangers (even the manager of the supermarket my dad was pilfering from).

Most people have been affected by this disease, either by knowing someone or caring for a loved one. They understand. Don't be embarrassed by the behaviors of your loved one who is in the throes of AD. Allow others to demonstrate their compassion toward you and your family. You will be surprised by how many will do just that.

FIND OUT NOW

My mother had herself convinced that she had AD. Rightfully so, considering our family history. I wasn't convinced her issues were AD related. If we had allowed this to result in a stalemate, if we had just stuck our head in the sand or dismissed her concerns or avoided a diagnosis out of fear, we would have never known that some of her issues were not AD and could be treated. You've heard Marwan stress the importance of this. Early intervention makes a huge difference. So please, don't put off the visit to your physician or neurologist.

NO ONE-SIZE-FITS-ALL FOR CAREGIVERS

As much as I would have liked my stepmother, Jane, to seek out support to help her deal with my father, that was not something she felt comfortable with. You, too, may be at odds with one of your family members on the direction of treatment for a loved one with AD.

That's okay. There is nothing to gain by pushing someone to do something they are resistant to. Do your best to be supportive, and remember that sometimes a hug is all it takes to help someone get through the day.

As we discussed in our last chapter, caregiving is a tough job, and all those involved need to offer one another a little breathing room and a lot of patience.

VOLUNTEER!

Volunteers are the backbone of research. And yet, 80 percent of AD studies are unable to meet their recruitment goals. There are many reasons for this, but here's what I will say. Doing it, volunteering yourself or your loved one for studies is not only altruistic, it's a fantastic strategic plan. You will have your finger on the pulse of what is new. You will learn a great deal, as I have. You will feel like you are part of the solution, not the problem. From the first time I participated in the study at Banner, I began to feel less like a victim and more like a fighter. I'm still part of that longitudinal study and proud of it! Again, without those of us participating in these studies, there would be no research, and there will be no cure.

Join us! Information on how you or a family member can become research volunteers is included in our resource guide at the end of this book.

HOLD ONTO FAITH

Many times through this journey I have been challenged, enduring pain and anxiety that sometimes seemed unsurmountable. My faith was part of what got me through it. It prevented me from leaving this world, knowing that my experience was given to me to make a difference, to leave a valuable imprint when I'm no longer here. That faith also helped me realize that instead of a genetic death sentence, I'd actually been given a gift. Today, I wake up every morning knowing I have a purpose in life.

LEARN TO LOVE AGAIN

Alzheimer's taught me we all are human, and we all have our imperfections that sometimes hurt others. In my case, it allowed me to see my father in a way I never imagined. The harsh, angry, and insensitive man I perceived in my childhood became a very different person. When I finally was able to look into those empty eyes, I saw my own imperfect reflection of myself. Yes, I could love him and myself again.

YOUR VOICE IS IMPORTANT

As you've read in my story, it took me quite a while to discover my voice. I have been silenced many times in the past, but now I'm being invited to use my voice. Whether it has been speaking at the American Association of Neurologists, to our representatives in Washington, to the media, or through the pages of this book, I feel now that my words are no longer falling on deaf ears.

I think back to the night a few years ago when I saw Helen Reddy onstage as part of the San Diego reading of Trish Vradenburg's play, *Surviving Grace*. I felt that my true self was embodied in Helen's iconic lyrics, "I am woman, hear me roar."

In my own polite way, I'm still roaring about the disease that ravaged my family and so many others, and that may eventually take me too.

But I'll tell you this. I'm not going down without a fight.

Appendix I

DR. SABBAGH

I'm a researcher in a fast-changing field of medicine. In this book, I've referred to important new studies on AD. But in order to better understand and appreciate the significance of these studies—as well as future studies you may see reported in the news media—it's important to recognize that there are many different types of investigations that we researchers undertake. Here's a brief rundown on some of the most common types.

OBSERVATIONAL STUDIES

All studies seek to address a hypothesis, a scientific question. One way to test a hypothesis is through observational studies. In observational studies, people go about their daily lives as they choose. They exercise when they want, eat what they like, and take the medicines their health-care providers prescribe. Participants report these activities to researchers. Researchers will gather all kinds of data about the people they are studying. In the example above, they will gather blood pressures on the participants and determine if people with high blood pressure are having more strokes—or strokes more often—than people with normal blood pressure. However, there are variables that need to be accounted for, including physical activity, diabetes, heart disease, obesity, and others.

Thus, making a connection between blood pressure and stroke is not as simple as it sounds. In an observational study, there is no intervention or treatment. But these types of studies are informative and in many cases are easier to conduct than randomized clinical trials.

RANDOMIZED CONTROLLED TRIALS

Randomized controlled trials are considered the gold standard for studying new treatments. Similar to cohort studies, randomized trials follow people over time and are expensive to do. Because participants are randomly assigned to an intervention (like a new drug or exercise) or standard treatment, these studies are more likely to show the true link between an intervention and a health outcome (like survival). Using the example above, a clinical trial would test whether taking a blood pressure medication on a regular basis would reduce the frequency of strokes over time.

For example, in a randomized controlled trial of a drug to remove amyloid and AD, researchers might assign half of the participants to a new drug to treat Alzheimer's and half to a placebo. If at the end of the study, the people on the study drug were better in terms of memory or function than the placebo group, the drug would be considered efficacious. Many behaviors, like altering smoking or alcohol drinking habits, cannot be tested in this way because it would not be ethical to assign people to a behavior known to be harmful. In these cases, researchers must use observational studies.

CASE-CONTROL STUDIES

Case-control studies are easy and fairly inexpensive to conduct, but they have pros and cons. They are a good way for researchers to study rare diseases and diseases that take a long time to develop. If a disease is rare, you would need to follow a large group of people long enough to have many cases of the disease develop. Since case-control studies look at past exposures of people who already have a disease, they are a good way to study such diseases, but there are potential problems. First, it can be hard for people to remember details about the past, especially when it comes to things like diet. Second, memories can be biased (or influenced) by the fact that the information is gathered after an event (like the diagnosis of ApoE4). Third, when it comes to sensitive topics (like drugs and alcohol), people with the disease may be much more likely to give complete information about their history than the control group (the people without the disease). Such differences in reporting can impact the accuracy of the results of case-control studies.

PROSPECTIVE COHORT STUDIES

A prospective cohort study follows a large group of people for a period of time. Some people will be exposed to something (like exercise) and others will not. Researchers compare the different groups to see which group is more likely to develop an outcome (such as AD). For example, they might compare people who exercise every day to those who work out three times a week and sedentary people.

ANIMAL STUDIES

Animal studies add to researchers' understanding of how and why some factors cause diseases in people. However, animal studies, such as those done with mice or rats, are designed differently from human studies. First, they will genetically engineer the animals to reproduce the disease in question. The animals usually have an accelerated form of the disease and a short life span (two years). Scientists then use these animals to test drugs to address specific diseases. They often look at exposures in larger doses and for shorter durations than are suitable for people. While animal studies can be helpful for future research in people, be wary of conclusions that are made from these studies. In almost every single study of drugs first applied in animal models, the drug showed success and efficacy that were subsequently not reproduced in humans. Thus, human populations need human studies.[1]

Appendix 2

LIFESTYLE, COGNITIVE TRAINING, AND HEART AND WEIGHT MONITORING STUDY

The Finnish Geriatric Intervention Study to Prevent Cognitive Impairment and Disability (FINGER), conducted by the Alzheimer's Research and Prevention Foundation, was the first randomized-controlled trial (RCT) for people like Jamie with the ApoE4 gene who are at risk for AD.

In this study published in the *Lancet* in 2015, people were randomly selected to receive one of several clinical interventions. A control group is one that is either given no intervention or, in the case of a drug study, gets a placebo, such as a sugar pill. The subjects who are given interventions (or medications) are then compared to those who were not to see if they've had any real effect. This landmark study, which had nearly 1,300 participants, ages sixty to seventy-seven, and spanned two years, found ways to prevent cognitive impairment; decrease cardiovascular risk factors, disability, and depression; and generally improve a dementia patient's quality of life. No small feat!

Many of the interventions successfully used in FINGER were already recommended practices before the results were published, yet the FINGER study confirms the validity of these recommendations. Moreover, subsequent studies have confirmed the FINGER results, which showed significant benefits in overall cognitive performance. The protective factors against cognitive decline, according to the study, are dietary guidance, physical activity, cognitive training, social activity, and intensive monitoring and management by a clinician of metabolic and cardiovascular risk factors. Later, we will talk these through one-by-one.

DIET AND WEIGHT
MANAGEMENT PROTOCOL

The protocol for this study was developed by Dale Bredesen, MD, with affiliations with UCLA School of Medicine and the Buck Institute, which he calls the Metabolic Enhancement for NeuroDegeneration (MEND). The MEND protocol confirms the FINGER recommendations for diet and weight management. In addition to what and how much you eat, the MEND study shows it is important to regulate how often. The technical term for this is *autophagy*. MEND found that going twelve to fourteen hours between your last meal (tantamount to modest fasting daily) and your first meal of the day will have a beneficial effect on your brain. (This means no raiding the refrigerator at night because it will spike your insulin.) The added value is that we go into a mild ketonic state when we fast for twelve hours, which can have benefits on the brain. The June 2016 issue of *Aging*, which published an updated version of the MEND study, found that out of ten participants with either "well-defined mild cognitive impairment, subjective cognitive impairment, or frank Alzheimer's disease diagnosis" prior to beginning the program, nine improved. Some were able to go back to work. Others regained mathematic skills. The MEND protocol included more than two dozen interventions (multimodal interventions), including a gluten-free diet, yoga, or another form of mindfulness practice, and a number of natural agents such as curcumin, fish oil, vitamin D, correcting vitamin deficiencies, normalizing sleep, correcting thyroid dysfunction, physical exercise, and others. This anecdotal case series, not conducted as a randomized study, caught the imagination of the general public and is now being sought by many.

But the most significant factor, in Dr. Bredesen's view, was a requirement to fast at least three hours before sleep and at least twelve hours between evening and morning meals. Dr. Bredesen acknowledges that most patients would have difficulty following everything in his protocol and that his study is small compared with FINGER, which had more than a thousand subjects. Additionally, there are no long-term objective studies supporting the results from the original case study of these ten subjects. Still, Dr. Bredesen's findings certainly give researchers in the field, like me, food for thought and, based on its merit, an interest in seeing more data.[1]

MULTI-INTERVENTION LIFESTYLE STUDY WITH NUTRITIONAL COUNSELING

Another clinical trial that shows the benefits in lifestyle changes is the Multidomain Alzheimer Preventive Trial (MAPT). This large, long-term trial is specifically designed to test whether multiple interventions consisting of nutritional counseling, physical exercise, and cognitive stimulation in combination with omega-3 fatty acid supplementation is effective in slowing cognitive decline in older adults at risk of AD.

The idea behind the study is that multiple interventions are likely to be more beneficial than a single intervention. This approach has another advantage; the interventions tested are widely available to millions of older adults. Additionally, MAPT includes studies to investigate beta-amyloid and the potential impact multidomain intervention and/or omega-3 supplementation has on cerebral metabolism and the rate of brain atrophy (shrinkage). More follow-up needs to be done but, once again, lifestyle changes, including diet and exercise, are proven to be essential for keeping Alzheimer's disease in check, especially for those who are high risk.[2]

HIGH RISK STUDY FOR APOE4

Jamie is participating in GeneMatch, a national program that recruits participants for Alzheimer's prevention studies using genetic testing (www.endalznow.org/study-opportunities/genematch).

As explained on the website of the Alzheimer's Prevention Registry, this program—which is hosted by Banner Alzheimer's Institute, in partnership with a number of other major research institutions—helps scientists find qualified participants for studies. The lack of subjects is an issue in Alzheimer's research. As the Registry notes, 80 percent of research studies don't complete enrollment on time because they can't recruit enough volunteers. This important program is helping to change that.

The Generation Program is made up of two clinical trials: Generation Study 1 and Generation Study 2. The GeneMatch registry can help with the recruitment for the Generation studies.

These studies are not looking for people with Alzheimer's but rather those with a specific form of the ApoE4 gene that can increase the risk of developing the disease.[3]

The goal of the Generation Program is to find out whether experimental medications can prevent the onset of Alzheimer's symptoms. In these clinical trials, researchers will test the study medications against a placebo. Research shows a link between a substance called amyloid beta and Alzheimer's disease. The study medications may stop amyloid beta from building up in the brain. Participants in this program could advance doctors' understanding of how to potentially prevent the onset of Alzheimer's.[4]

Participants in the Generation 2 study, who are between sixty and seventy-five, already know by choice or by accident that they are carriers of the ApoE4 gene. If you don't know whether or not you are a carrier of the gene (and you want to know), the researchers will put you in touch with GeneMatch, which will mail you a DNA cheek-swab test kit. The idea behind the Generation study is to see if you have higher than expected levels of amyloid in your brain because you carry the ApoE4. By finding people at high risk with amyloid, subjects will then have the option to receive treatments before the symptoms appear. When ordering a swab test by mail, you will not be told your results unless you are invited to a study site.[5]

SWEDISH STUDY CONFIRMS INTERVENTIONS WORK FOR APOE4 CARRIERS

As I mentioned previously in the FINGER study section, subjects between sixty and seventy-seven years old with risk factors for memory disorders were divided into two groups. One was given regular-lifestyle counseling only and the other enhanced-lifestyle counseling that involved nutrition advice, physical and cognitive exercises, and support in managing the risk of cardiovascular diseases. Findings revealed that the regular-lifestyle-counseling group had a significantly increased risk of cognitive and functional decline compared to the group that engaged in lifestyle interventions. In 2018, Swedish researchers followed up on the results of the FINGER study to see if the presence of the ApoE4 gene affected the intervention results. The study group had a total of 1,109 people, 362 of whom were carriers of the ApoE4 gene. The findings showed that enhanced-lifestyle counseling prevented cognitive decline in those with the risk gene. According to the Swedish study, people with

ApoE4 responded as well or better than those subjects who do not have the gene.[6]

"Many people worry that genetic risk factors for dementia may thwart potential benefits from healthy lifestyle changes," said adjunct professor Alina Solomon, the lead author of the study in *Science Daily*. "We were very happy to see that this was not the case in our intervention, which was started early, before the onset of substantial cognitive impairment." Professor Miia Kivipelto, principal investigator of the FINGER trial, added, "The FINGER intervention model is now being adapted and tested globally in the World Wide FINGERS initiative. New clinical trials in diverse populations with a variety of geographical and cultural backgrounds will help us formulate global dementia prevention strategies." Studies like these show that it may be possible to win the tug-of-war against your genes, and using lifestyle changes, such as diet, exercise, and restorative sleep, is an evidence-based way to do that.[7]

MONITORING GENE MUTATIONS FOR AD

Please be aware that the following only applies to just a few people in the world, but it's important to see the full picture of where AD research is.

An observational study was performed that enabled researchers around the world to monitor and identify changes in individuals who carry one of the gene mutations (Presenilin1, Presenilin2 or APP) known to cause what's called "dominantly inherited Alzheimer's disease." These are rare mutations handed down generation after generation. While individuals like Jamie have a 91 percent chance of getting AD by virtue of their 4/4 status, a few people have even rarer mutations bumping their chances of getting the disease to 100 percent. I do this for a living, and I think I diagnose a patient with dominantly inherited Alzheimer's disease once a decade.

The Dominantly Inherited Alzheimer Network (DIAN) trial evaluated participants with clinical and cognitive testing, brain imaging, and biological fluid collection (blood, cerebrospinal fluid) with the goal of determining changes in presymptomatic gene carriers who are destined to develop AD. Another goal is to establish a research database and tissue repository to support research by other investigators around the world. Knowledge gained from this long-term study may lead to therapeutic options to detect and treat AD at its earliest stage or prevent it all together.[8]

Resource Guide

H ere is a guide to sources for getting involved in research and clinical trials, plus a state-by-state listing of Alzheimer's Disease Research Centers around the country. For a comprehensive and updated guide on all aspects of the disease, including detailed information on everything from financial and legal assistance to grief counseling, visit www.alzbabes.org.

RESEARCH AND CLINICAL TRIAL INFORMATION

A-LIST: ALIST4RESEARCH.ORG

The A-List is the collective voice of those living with Alzheimer's and other dementias, at-risk adults, caregivers, and families who demand that their preferences are heard and respected by the research community.

ALZHEIMER'S PREVENTION REGISTRY: ENDALZNOW.ORG

Led by Banner Alzheimer's Institute, this registry unites leading researchers with people who are interested in taking part in Alzheimer's studies.

GENEMATCH: ENDALZNOW.ORG/GENEMATCH

This site connects Alzheimer's prevention studies with genetic testing through free cheek-swab kits to match volunteers with research opportunities.

RESOURCE GUIDE

BEING PATIENT: BEINGPATIENT.COM

Being Patient is an editorially independent news site covering the latest Alzheimer's research.

BRAIN HEALTH REGISTRY: BRAINHEALTHREGISTRY.ORG

This registry recruits and observes people who answer online questions (health, lifestyle, and medical history) and take online brain tests. The goal is to build a large pool of potential research participants for clinical trials, reducing the time and cost of research.

NATIONAL INSTITUTE ON AGING: NIA.NIH.GOV/ALZHEIMERS/

Find NIA/NIH clinical trials and studies related to Alzheimer's, other dementias, mild cognitive impairment, and caregiving. (Also see the Alzheimer's Disease Research Center section of this guide.)

TRIALMATCH: TRIALMATCH.ALZ.ORG

The Alzheimer's Association's TrialMatch is a clinical trial matching service that generates customized lists of studies based on user-provided information.

ALZHEIMER'S DISEASE RESEARCH CENTER DIRECTORY (NIA/NIH)

———— ARIZONA ————

ARIZONA ALZHEIMER'S CONSORTIUM
Eric Reiman, MD, Director
Arizona Alzheimer's Disease Center
Banner Alzheimer's Institute
901 E. Willeta Street
Phoenix, AZ 85006
Website: http://azalz.org/

Information line: 602-839-6900
Director's e-mail: eric.reiman@bannerhealth.com
Director's phone: 602-839-6999
Fax: 602-839-6253

——— CALIFORNIA ———

STANFORD ALZHEIMER'S DISEASE RESEARCH CENTER
Stanford University
Victor W. Henderson, MD, MS, Director
259 Campus Drive, MC 5405
Stanford, CA 94305–5405
Website: med.stanford.edu/adrc.html
Information line: 650-721-2409
ADRC e-mail: adrcstanford@stanford.edu
Director's e-mail: vhenderson@stanford.edu
Director's phone: 650-723-5456
Fax: 650-725-6591

UC DAVIS ALZHEIMER'S DISEASE CENTER
University of California, Davis Medical Center
Charles S. DeCarli, MD, Director
4860 Y Street, Suite 3700
Sacramento, CA 95817–4540
Website: www.ucdmc.ucdavis.edu/alzheimers
Information line: 916-734-5496
Director's e-mail: cdecarli@ucdmc.ucdavis.edu
Director's phone: 916-734-8413
Fax: 916-734-6525

UC DAVIS SATELLITE CENTER
UC Davis East Bay
100 North Wiget Lane, Suite 150

Walnut Creek, CA 94598
John Olichney, MD, Director
Director's phone: 925-357-6515
Director's e-mail: jmolichney@ucdavis.edu

UC IRVINE
Frank LaFerla, PhD, Director
Alzheimer's Disease Research Center
University of California, Irvine
5120 Natural Sciences II
Irvine, CA 92697
Website: www.mind.uci.edu
Information line: 949-824-3253
Director's e-mail: laferla@uci.edu
Director's phone: 949-824-5315
Fax: 949-824-2447

UC SAN DIEGO
James Brewer, MD, PhD, Director
Alzheimer's Disease Research Center
University of California, San Diego
9500 Gilman Drive (0948)
La Jolla, CA 92093–0948
Website: http://adrc.ucsd.edu
Information line: 858-822-4800
ADRC e-mail: adrc@ucsd.edu
Director's e-mail: jbrewer@ucsd.edu
Fax: 858-247-1287

UC SAN DIEGO SATELLITE CENTER
UC San Diego Hispanic Satellite and Outreach
9444 Medican Center Drive, Suite 1–100
La Jolla, CA 92037

James Brewer, MD, PhD, Director
Center phone: 858-822-4800
Director's e-mail: jbrewer@ucsd.edu

UC SAN FRANCISCO
Bruce L. Miller, MD, Director
Alzheimer's Disease Research Center
University of California, San Francisco Memory and Aging Center
675 Nelson Rising Lane, Suite 190
San Francisco, CA 94158
Website: http://memory.ucsf.edu
Information line: 415-476-3722
ADRC e-mail: adrc@memory.ucsf.edu
Director's e-mail: bmiller@memory.ucsf.edu
Director's phone: 415-476-5591
Fax: 415-476-4800

UNIVERSITY OF SOUTHERN CALIFORNIA
Helena Chui, MD, Director
Alzheimer's Disease Research Center
University of Southern California
1540 Alcazor Street, CHP, Suite 215
Los Angeles, CA 90033
Website: http://adrc.usc.edu
Information line: 323-442-7600
ADRC e-mail: askadrc@usc.edu
Director's e-mail: chui@usc.edu
Director's phone: 323-442-7686
Fax: 323-442-7689

RESOURCE GUIDE

—— CONNECTICUT ——

YALE UNIVERSITY
Stephen Strittmatter, MD, PhD, Director
Yale University Alzheimer's Disease Center
295 Congress Avenue, BCMM 4368
PO Box 9812
New Haven, CT 06536
Website: http://medicine.yale.edu/adrc
Center e-mail: adrc@yale.edu
Information line: 203-785-4736
Director's phone: 203-785-4878
Fax: 203-785-5098
Director's e-mail: stephen.strittmatter@yale.edu

—— FLORIDA ——

MAYO CLINIC, JACKSONVILLE
Neill Graff-Radford, MD, Associate Director
Memory Disorder Clinic
4500 San Pablo Road
Jacksonville, FL 32224
Website: www.mayo.edu/research/centers-programs/
alzheimers-disease-research-center
Center phone: 904-953-6523

UNIVERSITY OF FLORIDA ALZHEIMER'S DISEASE CENTER
Todd E. Golde, MD, PhD, Director
1Florida Alzheimer's Disease Research Center

University of Florida
Center for Translational Research in Neurodegenerative Disease
1275 Center Drive
BMS J-497
PO Box 100159
Gainesville, FL 32610–0159
Website: http://1floridaadrc.org
Center e-mail: info@1floridaadrc.org
Information line: 352-273-7436
Director's e-mail: tgolde@ufl.edu
Director's phone: 352-273-9456
Fax: 352-294-5060

—— GEORGIA ——

EMORY UNIVERSITY
Allan I. Levey, MD, PhD, Director
Alzheimer's Disease Center
Neurology Department
Emory Brain Health Center
12 Executive Park Drive
Atlanta, GA 30329
Website: http://alzheimers.emory.edu
Information line: 404-712-6838
ADRC e-mail: emoryadrc@emory.edu
Director's e-mail: alevey@emory.edu
Director's phone: 404-727-7220
Fax: 404-727-3999

—— ILLINOIS ——

NORTHWESTERN UNIVERSITY
M. Marsel Mesulam, MD, Director

Cognitive Neurology and Alzheimer's Disease Center
Feinberg School of Medicine
Northwestern University
675 North St. Claire, Galter 20–100
Chicago, IL 60611
Website: www.brain.northwestern.edu
Information line: 312-926-1851
Director's e-mail: mmesulam@northwestern.edu
Director's phone: 312-908-9339
Fax: 312-908-8789

Rush University Medical Center
Alzheimer's Disease Center
David A. Bennett, MD, Director
Armour Academic Center
600 South Paulina Street, Suite 1028
Chicago, IL 60612
Website: www.rush.edu/services/alzheimers-disease-center
Information line: 312-942-3333
Director's e-mail: david_a_bennett@rush.edu
Director's phone: 312-942-2362
Fax: 312-563-4605

——— INDIANA ———

Indiana University
Andrew Saykin, PsyD, Director
Indiana Alzheimer Disease Center
IU Health Neuroscience Center
Indiana University School of Medicine
355 West 16th Street, Suite 4100
Indianapolis, IN 46202
Website: http://iadc.medicine.iu.edu

Information line: 317-963-7599

ADRC e-mail: iadc@iu.edu

Director's e-mail: asaykin@iu.edu

Director's phone: 317-963-7501

Fax: 317-963-7547

IU SATELLITE CENTER

Healthy Aging Brain Center

Sandra Eskenazi Center for Brain Care Innovation

Malaz A. Boustani, MD, Director

Eskenazi Health

720 Eskenazi Avenue

Indianapolis, Indiana 46202

Website: http://brain.eskenazihealth.edu/sandra

Center phone: 317-880-2224

Director's e-mail: mboustan@iu.edu

—— KANSAS ——

UNIVERSITY OF KANSAS

Russell H. Swerdlow, MD, Director

Alzheimer's Disease Center

University of Kansas

3091 Rainbow Boulevard

Mail Stop 6002

Kansas City, KS 66160

Website: www.kualzheimer.org

Information line: 913-588-0555

ADRC e-mail: kuamp@kumc.edu

Director's e-mail: rswerdlow@kumc.edu

Director's phone: 913-945-6632

Fax: 913-945-5035

KENTUCKY

UNIVERSITY OF KENTUCKY
Linda Van Eldik, PhD, Director
University of Kentucky Alzheimer's Disease Center
Sanders-Brown Center on Aging
101 Sanders-Brown Building
800 South Limestone Street
Lexington, KY 40536–0230
Website: www.uky.edu/coa
Information line: 859-323-6040
Director's e-mail: linda.vaneldik@uky.edu
Director's phone: 859-257-5566
Fax: 859-323-2866

UK SATELLITE CENTER
Minority Gateway Clinic
Charles D. Smith, MD, Director
UK Polk Dalton Clinic
217 Elm Tree Lane
Lexington, KY 40507
Center phone: 859-323-5550
Director's e-mail: csmith@mri.uky.edu

MARYLAND

JOHNS HOPKINS UNIVERSITY
Marilyn Albert, PhD, Director
Alzheimer's Disease Research Center
Johns Hopkins University
Reed Hall 226
1620 McElderry Street

Baltimore, MD 21205
Website: www.alzresearch.org
Information line: 410-502-5164
Director's e-mail: malbert9@jhmi.edu
Director's phone: 410-614-3040
Fax: 410-502-2189

——— MASSACHUSETTS ———

BOSTON UNIVERSITY
Neil Kowall, MD, Director
Alzheimer's Disease Center
Boston VA Medical Center
Neurology Service C-1271
150 South Huntington Avenue
Jamaica Plain, MA 02130
Website: www.bu.edu/alzresearch
Information line: 1–888-458-2823
ADRC e-mail: buad@bu.edu
Director's e-mail: nkowall@bu.edu
Director's phone: 857-364-4831
Fax: 857-364-4454

MASSACHUSETTS GENERAL HOSPITAL /
HARVARD MEDICAL SCHOOL
Bradley T. Hyman, MD, PhD, Director
Alzheimer's Disease Research Center
Massachusetts General Hospital
Department of Neurology
CNY 114–2009
16th Street
Charlestown, MA 02129

Website: http://madrc.org
Information line: 617-726-3987
Director's e-mail: bhyman@partners.org
Director's phone: 617-726-2299
Fax: 617-724-1480

—— MICHIGAN ——

UNIVERSITY OF MICHIGAN
Henry Paulson, MD, PhD, Director
University of Michigan Alzheimer's Disease Center
2101 Commonwealth Boulevard, Suite D
Ann Arbor, MI 48105
Website: http://alzheimers.med.umich.edu
Information line: 734-936-8803
Director's e-mail: henryp@med.umich.edu
Director's phone: 734-615-5632
Fax: 734-764-6444

—— MINNESOTA ——

MAYO CLINIC
Ronald C. Petersen, MD, PhD, Director
Alzheimer's Disease Research Center
Department of Neurology
200 1st Street S.W.
Rochester, MN 55905
Website: www.mayo.edu/research/centers-programs/
alzheimers-disease-research-center
Information line: 507-284-1324
ADRC e-mail: mayoadc@mayo.edu
Director's e-mail: peter8@mayo.edu

Director's phone: 507-538-0487
Director's fax: 507-538-6012
Main fax: 507-538-0878

———— MISSOURI ————

WASHINGTON UNIVERSITY IN ST. LOUIS
John C. Morris, MD, Director
Alzheimer's Disease Research Center
Washington University School of Medicine
Department of Neurology
4488 Forest Park Avenue, Suite 130
St. Louis, MO 63110
Website: http://alzheimer.wustl.edu
Information line: 314-286-2683
Director's e-mail: morrisj@abraxas.wustl.edu
Director's phone: 314-286-2881
Fax: 314-286-2763

———— NEW YORK ————

COLUMBIA UNIVERSITY
Scott Small, MD, Director
Columbia University Alzheimer's Disease Center
Sergievsky Center
630 West 168th Street, PH 18
New York, NY 10032
Website: www.cumc.columbia.edu/adrc
Information line: 212-305-9168
Director's e-mail: sas68@columbia.edu
Director's phone: 212-305-1269
Fax: 212-342-4554

RESOURCE GUIDE

COLUMBIA U. SATELLITE CENTER
ADRC Northern Manhattan Community Satellite
Memory Disorders, 1st Floor
Lawrence S. Honig, MD, PhD, Director
1051 Riverside Drive
New York, NY 10032
Information line: 212-305-9168
E-mail: am4717@cumc.columbia.edu
Director's e-mail: lh456@cumc.columbia.edu

MOUNT SINAI SCHOOL OF MEDICINE
Mary Sano, PhD, Director
Alzheimer's Disease Research Center
Department of Psychiatry
Mount Sinai School of Medicine
One Gustave Levy Place, Box 1230
New York, NY 10029
Website: http://icahn.mssm.edu/research/adrc
Information line: 212-241-8329
Director's e-mail: mary.sano@mssm.edu
Director's phone: 718-741-4228
Fax: 718-562-9120

NEW YORK UNIVERSITY
Thomas Wisniewski, MD, Director
NYU Alzheimer's Disease Center
Center for Cognitive Neurology
145 E. 32nd Street, 5th Floor
New York, NY 10016
Website: www.med.nyu.edu/adc
Information line: 212-263-8088
Director's e-mail: thomas.wisniewski@nyumc.org

Director's phone: 212-263-3252

Fax: 212-263-6991

NYU Satellite Center

Alzheimer's Disease Center Multicultural Program

Karyn Marsh, PhD, Director

New York University

Langone Medical Center

145 East 32nd Street, 2nd Floor

New York, NY 11216

Center phone: 212-263-3201

Director's e-mail: karyn.marsh@nyumc.org

———— NORTH CAROLINA ————

Wake Forest University

Suzanne Craft, PhD, Director

Wake Forest Alzheimer's Disease Core Center

Wake Forest School of Medicine

Internal Medicine, Geriatrics and Gerontology

Medical Center Boulevard

Winston Salem, NC 27157–0001

Website: www.wakehealth.edu/alzheimers/

Information line: 336–716-MIND (6463) or 855–381-MIND (6463)

Director's E-mail: suzcraft@wakehealth.edu

Director's phone: 336-713-8830

Fax: 336-713-8826

———— OREGON ————

Oregon Health and Science University

Jeffrey Kaye, MD, Director

Aging and Alzheimer's Disease Center CR 131
3181 SW Sam Jackson Park Road
Portland, OR 97239–3098
Website: http://www.ohsu.edu/xd/health/services/brain/getting-
treatment/diagnosis/alzheimers-aging-dementia/index.cfm
Information line: 503-494-6976
Director's e-mail: kaye@ohsu.edu
Director's phone: 503-494-6976
Fax: 503-494-7499

——— PENNSYLVANIA ———

UNIVERSITY OF PENNSYLVANIA
John Q. Trojanowski, MD, PhD, Director
Alzheimer's Disease Center
3rd Floor Maloney
3600 Spruce Street
Philadelphia, PA 19104–4283
Website: http://pennmemorycenter.org
Information line: 215-662-7810
Director's e-mail: trojanow@mail.med.upenn.edu
Director's phone: 215-662-6399
Fax: 215-349-5909

UNIVERSITY OF PITTSBURGH
Oscar Lopez, MD, Director
Alzheimer's Disease Research Center
Department of Neurology
3501 Forbes Avenue, Suite 830
Pittsburgh, PA 15213
Website: www.adrc.pitt.edu
Information line: 412-692-2700

Director's e-mail: lopezol@upmc.edu
Director's phone: 412-246-6869
Center's fax: 412-246-6873

UNIVERSITY OF PITTSBURGH SATELLITE CENTER

Alzheimer's Outreach and Resource Center
Hill House Association
Oscar Lopez, MD, Director
1835 Centre Avenue, Suite 230
Pittsburgh, PA 15219
Center phone: 412-261-0742
Director's e-mail: lopezol@upmc.edu

———— TEXAS ————

UNIVERSITY OF TEXAS, SOUTHWESTERN MEDICAL CENTER

Roger N. Rosenberg, MD, Director
Alzheimer's Disease Research Center
University of Texas SW Medical Center
5323 Harry Hines Boulevard
Dallas, TX 75390–9129
Website: www.utsouthwestern.edu/education/medicalschool/departments/neurology/programs/alzeimers-disease-center
Information line: 214-648-0563
ADC e-mail: adc@utsouthwestern.edu
Director's e-mail: roger.rosenberg@utsouthwestern.edu
Director's phone: 214-648-3239
Fax: 214-648-6824

———— WASHINGTON ————

NATIONAL ALZHEIMER'S COORDINATING CENTER (NACC)

Walter Kukull, PhD, Director

National Alzheimer's Coordinating Center
4311 11th Avenue NE, Suite 300
Seattle, WA 98105
Website: www.alz.washington.edu
Information line: 206-543-8637
E-mail: naccmail@uw.edu
Fax: 206-616-5927

UNIVERSITY OF WASHINGTON
Thomas Grabowski, MD, Director
Alzheimer's Disease Research Center
University of Washington
Box 357115
Seattle, WA 98195–7115
Website: www.pathology.washington.edu/research/adrc
Information line: 855-744-0588
ADRC e-mail: uwadrc@uw.edu
Director's e-mail: tgrabow@uw.edu
Director's phone: 206-616-0021
Fax: 206-543-3495

——— WISCONSIN ———

UNIVERSITY OF WISCONSIN
Sanjay Asthana, MD, Director
Wisconsin Alzheimer's Disease Research Center
University of Wisconsin
2870 University Avenue, Suite 106
Madison, WI 53705
Website: www.adrc.wisc.edu
Information line: 608-263-2582
ADRC e-mail: adrc@medicine.wisc.edu
Director's e-mail: sa@medicine.wisc.edu

RESOURCE GUIDE

Director's phone: 608-262-8597 or 608-263-9969
Fax: 608-280-7165

UNIVERSITY OF WISCONSIN SATELLITE CENTER
Wisconsin ADRC Minority Recruitment Satellite Program
Dorothy Edwards, PhD, Director
J5/1 Mezzanine
600 Highland Avenue
Madison, WI 53792
Center phone: 608-263-2582
Director's e-mail: dfedwards@education.wisc.edu

Notes

Chapter 2: The Devastating News

1. "What Causes Alzheimer's Disease?" National Institute on Aging, accessed October 13, 2018, https://www.nia.nih.gov/health /what-causes-alzheimers-disease/.

Chapter 4: The ABCs of ALZ

1. Hanns Hippius and Gabriele Nuendörfer, "The Discovery of Alzheimer's Disease," *Dialogues in Clinical Neuroscience*, 5, no. 1 (March 2003): 101–108, https://www.ncbi.nlm.nih.gov/pmc/articles/PMC3181715/.

2. Robert Katzman, "The Prevalence and Malignancy of Alzheimer's Disease," *Archives of Neurology* 33, no.4 (April 1976): 217–18, https://doi .org/10.1001/archneur.1976.00500040001001.

3. H. Roger Segelken, "Robert Katzman, Alzheimer's Activist, Dies at 82," *The New York Times*, September 23, 2008, https://www.nytimes .com/2008/09/24/us/24katzman.html.

4. "Facts and Figures," Alzheimer's Association, accessed October 24, 2018, https://www.alz.org/facts/.

5. Marie Pasinski and Jodie Gould, *Beautiful Brain, Beautiful You* (Boston: Hyperion/Harvard University, 2011), 75.

6. Human Genome Project Information Archive 1990–2003, accessed

217

October 24, 2018, https://web.ornl.gov/sci/techresources/Human
_Genome/index.shtml.

CHAPTER 5: THE GENETIC PUZZLE OF AD
1. Human Genome Project Information Project Archive 1990–2003,
accessed October 24, 2018, https://web.ornl.gov/sci/techresources
/Human_Genome/index.shtml.

CHAPTER 6: TO TEST OR NOT TO TEST
1. "What Is Genetic Testing?" Genetics Home Reference, US National
Library of Medicine, accessed October 24, 2018, https://ghr.nlm.nih.gov
/primer/testing/genetictesting/.
2. "Huntington Disease," MedlinePlus, accessed October 24, 2018, https
://medlineplus.gov/ency/article/000770.htm.
3. "Genes," MedlinePlus, accessed October 24, 2018, https://medlineplus
.gov/ency/article/002371.htm.
4. "Genes and Human Disease," Genomic Resource Centre, World Health
Organization, accessed October 24, 2018, www.who.int/genomics
/public/geneticdiseases/en/index3.html.
5. "GeneMatch, a Program of the Alzheimer's Prevention Registry Online,"
Alzheimer's Prevention Library, accessed October 24, 2018, https://www
.endalznow.org/study-opportunities/genematch/.
6. Robert C. Green et al., "Disclosure of APOE Genotype for Risk of
Alzheimer's Disease," *New England Journal of Medicine* 361 (July 16,
2009): 245–54, https://doi.org/10.1056/NEJMoa0809578.
7. S. A. Bemelmans et al., "Psychological, Behavioral and Social Effects
of Disclosing Alzheimer's Disease Biomarkers to Research Participants:
A Systematic Review," *Alzheimer's Research and Therapy* 8, no. 1
(November 2016): 46, https://doi.org/10.1186/s13195-016-0212-z.
8. Eun Kyung Kim, "Richard Engel Shares Heartbreaking Story of Son's
Medical Journey," Today.com, January 30, 2018, https://www.today.com
/health/richard-engel-shares-son-s-battle-rett-syndrome-genetic-disorder
-t121898.

9. "One Little Boy's DNA Brings the Promise of a Healthy Tomorrow for Many," Jan and Dan Duncan Neurological Research Institute, accessed October 24, 2018, http://www.duncannri.org/.

10. Kim, "Richard Engel Shares."

11. Anna Almendrala, "Home Genetic Tests May Be Riddled with Errors, and Companies Aren't Keeping Track," *Huffington Post*, April 3, 2018, https://www.huffingtonpost.com/entry/home-genetic-test-false-positives_us_5ac27188e4b04646b6451c42.

12. Almendrala, "Home Genetic Tests."

13. Jeneen Interlandi, "Should You Try an At-Home Genetic Test?" *Consumer Reports,* April 02, 2018, https://www.consumerreports.org/genetic-testing/at-home-genetic-test-kits-what-you-need-to-know/.

CHAPTER 8: THE REAL RISKS OF ALZHEIMER'S

1. K. Hao et al., "Shared Genetic Etiology Underlying Alzheimer's Disease and Type 2 Diabetes," *Molecular Aspects of Medicine* 43–44 (Jun–Oct 2015): 66–76, https://doi.org/10.1016/j.mam.2015.06.006.

2. E. R. Mayeda, R. A. Whitmer, and K. Yaffe, "Diabetes and Cognition," *Clinics in Geriatric Medicine* 31, no. 1 (February 2015): 101–15, https://doi.org/10.1016/j.cger.2014.08.021.

3. "Type 2 Diabetes," Mayo Clinic, accessed October 24, 2018, www.mayoclinic.org/diseases-conditions/type-2-diabetes/diagnosis-treatment/drc-20351199/.

4. Rachel A. Whitmer, "The Epidemiology of Adiposity and Dementia," *Current Alzheimer Research* 4, no. 2 (2007): 117–22, https://doi.org/10.2174/156720507780362065.

5. Whitmer, "Epidemiology of Adiposity and Dementia."

6. Whitmer, "Epidemiology of Adiposity and Dementia."

7. Whitmer, "Epidemiology of Adiposity and Dementia."

8. "What Is Vascular Disease?" WebMD, accessed October 25, 2018, https://www.webmd.com/heart-disease/vascular-disease#1.

9. "What Is Ischemia?" WebMD, accessed October 25, 2018, https://www.webmd.com/heart-disease/what-is-ischemia#1.

10. Matthew Hoffman, "Picture of the Brain," WebMD, accessed October 25, 2018, https://www.webmd.com/brain/picture-of-the-brain#1.

11. "What Is a TIA?" WebMD, accessed October 25, 2018, https://www.webmd.com/stroke/what-is-tia#1.

12. Miia Kivipelto et al., "Risk Score for the Prediction of Dementia Risk in 20 Years Among Middle Aged People: A Longitudinal, Population-Based Study," *The Lancet Neurology* 5, no. 9 (September 2006): 735–41, https://doi.org/10.1016/S1474-4422(06)70537-3.

13. M. S. Beeri et al., "Coronary Artery Disease Is Associated with Alzheimer's Disease Neuropathology in ApoE4 Carriers," *Neurology* 66, no. 9 (May 2006): 1399–1404, https://doi.org/10.1212/01.wnl.0000210447.19748.0b.

14. "Preventing Cognitive Decline and Dementia: A Way Forward," The National Academies of Science, Engineering, and Medicine, June 22, 2017, http://nationalacademies.org/hmd/reports/2017/preventing-cognitive-decline-and-dementia-a-way-forward.aspx.

15. K. Takahata, H. Tabuchi, and M. Mimura, "Late-onset Neurodegenerative Diseases Following Traumatic Brain Injury: Chronic Traumatic Encephalopathy (CTE) and Alzheimer's Disease Secondary to TBI (AD-TBI)," *Brain and Nerve* 68, no. 7 (July 2016): 849–57, https://doi.org/10.11477/mf.1416200517.

16. M. N. Sabbagh et al., "Smoking Affects the Phenotype of Alzheimer Disease," *Neurology* 64, no. 7 (April 2005): 1301–1303, https://doi.org/10.1212/01.WNL.0000156912.54593.65.

17. M. Rusanen et al., "Heavy Smoking in Midlife and Long-Term Risk of Alzheimer Disease and Vascular Dementia," *Archives of Internal Medicine* 171, no. 4 (February 2011): 333–9, https://doi.org/10.1001/archinternmed.2010.393.

CHAPTER 10: BECOMING A CAREGIVER

1. "Caregiver Statistics: Demographics," Family Caregiver Alliance, accessed October 17, 2018, https://www.caregiver.org/caregiver-statistics-demographics/.

2. Daisy Urgiles, "Gene Wilder's Widow Shares Heartfelt Essay on His Battle with Alzheimer's," *Guideposts*, accessed October 17, 2018, https://www.guideposts.org/friends-and-family/caregiving/caregiver-burnout/gene-wilders-widow-shares-heartfelt-essay-on-his/.

3. "Alzheimer's Disease and Caregiving," Family Caregiver Alliance, accessed October 17, 2018, https://www.caregiver.org/alzheimers-disease-caregiving.

4. "Alzheimer's: Smoothing the Transition on Moving Day," Mayo Clinic, accessed October 17, 2018, https://www.mayoclinic.org/healthy-lifestyle/caregivers/in-depth/alzheimers/art-20046610?pg=2/.

5. "Alzheimer's," Mayo Clinic.

6. Philip Sherwell, "Judge Lost Husband to Alzheimer's—and Love," *The Telegraph*, January 27, 2008, https://www.telegraph.co.uk/news/uknews/1576716/Judge-lost-husband-to-Alzheimers-and-love.html.

7. "Taking Care of YOU: Self-Care for Family Caregivers," Family Caregiver Alliance, accessed October 17, 2018, https://www.caregiver.org/taking-care-you-self-care-family-caregivers.

8. "Taking Care of YOU," Family Caregiver Alliance.

CHAPTER 11: PROTECTING YOURSELF AGAINST AD, PART ONE: DIET

1. N. Scarmeas et al., "Mediterranean Diet and Risk for Alzheimer's Disease," *Annals of Neurology* 59, no. 6 (June 2006): 912–21, https://doi.org/10.1002/ana.20854.

2. M. C. Morris et al., "MIND Diet Associated with Reduced Incidence of Alzheimer's Disease," *Alzheimer's and Dementia* 11, no. 9 (September 2015): 1007–14, https://doi.org/10.1016/j.jalz.2014.11.009.

3. "Hidden in Plain Sight," SugarScience, University of California–San Francisco, accessed October 18, 2018, sugarscience.ucsf.edu/hidden-in-plain-sight/.

4. J. M. Walker and F. E. Harrison, "Shared Neuropathological Characteristics of Obesity, Type 2 Diabetes and Alzheimer's Disease:

Impacts on Cognitive Decline," *Nutrients* 7, no. 9 (September 2015): 7332–57, https://doi.org/10.3390/nu7095341.

5. C. C. Tangney et al., "Adherence to a Mediterranean-Type Dietary Pattern and Cognitive Decline in a Community Population," *American Journal of Clinical Nutrition* 93, no. 3 (March 2011): 601–7, https://doi.org/10.3945/ajcn.110.007369.

6. Marwan Sabbagh, "How Do Dietary Habits Influence Alzheimer's Risk," slide presentation, 2014.

7. Sabbagh, "How Do Dietary Habits."

8. Sabbagh, "How Do Dietary Habits."

9. Sabbagh, "How Do Dietary Habits."

10. Sabbagh, "How Do Dietary Habits."

11. Sabbagh, "How Do Dietary Habits."

12. P. Marambaud, H. Zhao, and P. Davies, "Resveratrol Promotes Clearance of Alzheimer's Disease Amyloid-beta Peptides," *Journal of Biological Chemistry* 280, no. 45 (November 2005): 37377–82, https://doi.org/10.1074/jbc.M508246200.

13. R. K. Dubey et al., "Resveratrol, a Red Wine Constituent, Blocks the Antimitogenic Effects of Estradiol on Human Female Coronary Artery Smooth Muscle Cells," *Journal of Clinical Endocrinology and Metabolism* 95, no. 9 (September 2010): E9–17, https://doi.org/10.1210/jc.2010-0460.

14. Dubey, "Resveratrol."

CHAPTER 12: PROTECTING YOURSELF AGAINST AD, PART TWO: PHYSICAL ACTIVITY

1. "Doctors Say Exercise Is the Best Medicine for Cognitive Impairment," Being Patient, accessed October 19, 2018, https://www.beingpatient.com/mild-cognitive-impairment-exercise/.

2. "44-Year Study Ties Midlife Fitness to Lower Dementia Risk," Alzforum, March 28, 2018, https://www.alzforum.org/news/research-news/44-year-study-ties-midlife-fitness-lower-dementia-risk/.

3. "Study: Exercise Is Good for All Brains," HT Health, *Herald-Tribune*, July 23, 2015, http://health.heraldtribune.com/2015/07/23 /study-exercise-is-good-for-all-brains/.

4. Light Watkins, *Bliss More: How to Succeed in Meditation Without Really Trying* (New York: Ballantine Books, 2018).

5. Sat Bir Singh Khalsa and Jodie Gould, *Your Brain on Yoga* (Boston: Harvard Health Publications, 2013), 17.

6. "Combatting Loneliness One Conversation at a Time," Jo Cox Loneliness, accessed November 14, 2018, https://www.jocoxloneliness .org/pdf/a_call_to_action.pdf.

7. "Combatting Loneliness," Jo Cox Loneliness.

8. Paula Span, "Loneliness Can Be Deadly for Elders; Friends Are the Antidote," *New York Times*, December 30, 2016, https://www.nytimes .com/2016/12/30/health/loneliness-elderly.html.

9. Ceylan Yeginsu, "UK Appoints a Minister for Loneliness," *New York Times*, January 17, 2018, https://www.nytimes.com/2018/01/17/world /europe/uk-britain-loneliness.html/.

10. Yeginsu, "UK Appoints a Minister for Loneliness."

11. Jiska Cohen-Mansfield et al., "The Value of Social Attributes of Stimuli for Promoting Engagement in Persons with Dementia," *Journal of Nervous and Mental Disease* 198, no. 8 (August 2010): 586–92, https ://doi.org/10.1097/NMD.0b013e3181e9dc76.

12. "Social Interaction," Healthy Brains, accessed October 25, 2018, https ://healthybrains.org/pillar-social/.

13. "Preventive Visit and Yearly Wellness Exams," Medicare.gov, accessed October 19, 2018, https://www.medicare.gov/coverage /preventive-visit-yearly-wellness-exams.

CHAPTER 13: A WORLD WITHOUT ALZHEIMER'S? YES!

1. "What Is the A4 Study?" The A4 Study, http://a4study.org/about/.

2. "Biomarker Qualification for Risk of Mild Cognitive Impairment (MCI) Due to Alzheimer's Disease (AD) and Safety and Efficacy

Evaluation of Pioglitazone in Delaying Its Onset (TOMMORROW),"
ClinicalTrials.gov, accessed October 19, 2018, https://clinicaltrials.gov
/ct2/show/NCT01931566.

3. "People with Dementia Benefit from Goal-Oriented Therapy,"
   University of Exeter, *ScienceDaily*, July 18, 2017, www.sciencedaily.com
   /releases/2017/07/170718084608.htm.

APPENDIX I: DR. SABBAGH

1. "Komen Perspectives—The Importance of Clinical Trials in Breast
   Cancer Treatment," Susan G. Komen, July 26, 2012, https://ww5.
   komen.org/KomenPerspectives/Komen-Perspectives---The-Importance
   -of-Clinical-Trials-in-Breast-Cancer-Treatment-(July-2012).html.

APPENDIX 2: LIFESTYLE, COGNITIVE TRAINING, AND HEART
AND WEIGHT MONITORING STUDY

1. John Weeks, "Integrative MEND Protocol for Reversing Alzheimer's
   Picked Up in *Aging* and by George Washington University," *Integrative
   Medicine: A Clinician's Journal* 15, no. 4 (August 2016): 24–26, https
   ://www.ncbi.nlm.nih.gov/pmc/articles/PMC4991646/.

2. B. Vellas et al., "MAPT Study: A Multidomain Approach for Preventing
   Alzheimer's Disease: Design and Baseline Data," *Journal of Prevention of
   Alzheimer's Disease* 1, no. 1 (June 2014): 13–22, https
   ://www.ncbi.nlm.nih.gov/pmc/articles/PMC4652787/.

3. "Generation Program—Multiple Sites," Alzheimer's Prevention Registry,
   accessed October 23, 2018, https://www.endalznow.org/studies
   /generation-program-multiple-sites.

4. E. M. Reiman et al., "Alzheimer's Prevention Initiative: A Plan to
   Accelerate the Evaluation of Presymptomatic Treatments," *Journal of
   Alzheimer's Disease* 26, no. 3 (2011):321–9, https://doi.org/10.3233
   /JAD-2011-0059.

5. "Generation Program," Alzheimer's Prevention Registry,
   accessed October 25, 2018, https://www.endalznow.org/studies
   /generation-program-multiple-sites.

6. University of Eastern Finland, "Lifestyle Changes Prevent Cognitive Decline Even in Genetically Susceptible Individuals," *Science Daily,* January 25, 2018, www.sciencedaily.com /releases/2018/01/180125101309.htm.

7. A. Solomon et al., "Effect of the Apolipoprotein E Genotype on Cognitive Change During a Multidomain Lifestyle Intervention: A Subgroup Analysis of a Randomized Clinical Trial," *JAMA Neurology* 75, no. 4 (April 2018): 462–70, https://doi.org/10.1001/jamaneurol .2017.4365.

8. J. C. Morris et al., "Developing an International Network for Alzheimer Research: The Dominantly Inherited Alzheimer Network," *Journal of Clinical Investigation* 2, no.10 (October 2012): 975–984, https://doi .org/10.4155/cli.12.93.

Acknowledgments

FROM JAMIE TYRONE:

First, my deepest thanks to Dr. Marwan Sabbagh for his belief in the importance of my story, and for giving me the courage and endurance to embark on a project that I never thought was possible. There were times when I questioned whether I was strong enough to continue. His patience and guidance are gifts I will forever cherish.

An unlimited amount of praise and thanks to our talented writer, John Hanc, who vividly brought my story to life and clearly articulated the complex genetic underpinnings of Alzheimer's, as well my coauthor's important insights into strategies for helping prevent and treat this disease.

My sincere appreciation to our literary agent, Linda Konner, who believed in this project, secured a publisher at lightning speed, and nurtured me through the process as a first time author. With gratitude to the masterful editors at HarperCollins Christian Publishing, Megan Dobson and Sam O'Neal; to writer Jodie Gould for her vital contributions to this project; and to Ann Napoletan, who create the fabulous and robust resource guide for the book and our website.

To my Banner Alzheimer's Institute family: Dr. Eric Reiman, Dr. Pierre Tariot, Jessica Langbaum, PhD, Dr. Richard Caselli with the Mayo Clinic, and the entire research team who constantly extend their gratitude for my research participation, and their tireless dedication to help find a cure.

To Dr. James Brewer, Dr. Doug Galasko, Lisa Delano-Wood, PhD, the team at the UCSD Shiley-Marcos Alzheimer's Disease Research Center, and to my earth angel Mary Sundsmo, who gave me a home and place of refuge when I needed it most.

To all genetic counselors that I love and revere, especially Susan Hahn, Susan Blanton, and Jill Goldman who gave me a platform, courage, and validation of my experience in order to use my voice.

To George Vradenburg and Meryl Comer, for having the confidence to invite me to be a founding member of WomenAgainstAlzheimer's—a network of USAgainstAlzheimer's. A special shout out to the hardworking team at USA2 who have given me the tools to be the advocate I am today. On behalf of all of us advocates, we thank you.

To research volunteers such as my friend Jeff Borghoff. You give the most precious gift to the fight against this disease: your time, dedication, and commitment. God bless every one of you.

To my gifted, kind, and compassionate therapist, Dr. Adrianne Ahern, who brought me from the brink of despair to embracing a bright and wonderful future. My heart sings every day.

To Carolyn Olsen, Jeanne Ames, Jeanne Irwin, Lynda Everman (the Energizer Babe), Marilyn Wotring, Rebecca Ailes-Fine, Jayne Slade, and Candice Berkman, all of whom allowed me to shed many tears followed by laughter and wonderful memories. Best Babes forever . . . .

To Doris Zallen, author of *To Test or Not to Test*, and Sally Sachar, whose writings prompted me to share my story to help others; to Donner Messner, Deborah Kan, and Julie Gregory, who have honored me by asking me for my opinions and suggestions.

To the G.O.L.D. Diggers (Gift of Loving Donors) who have been supportive with their continuous donations to B.A.B.E.S. from the very beginning. They warm my heart with their belief in my journey.

And finally, to my husband and the love of my life, Doug Tyrone. I hope that every reader of his book comes away knowing how witty, supportive, loving, and important you are in my life. I am one blessed girl.

FROM DR. MARWAN SABBAGH:

This manuscript was not written in a vacuum or in isolation. This is the handiwork of many, and they deserve to be acknowledged.

First, I wish to thank and acknowledge my coauthor, Jamie Tyrone. Without her story and her inspiration, there is no book to write.

Next, I wish to thank our agent, Linda Konner. Without her representation, I am not sure we would have gotten the traction needed to get this in front of our publisher.

Next, I wish to thank and acknowledge HarperCollins Christian Publishing. Sam O'Neal and Megan Dobson guided us masterfully through the publication process, and we are grateful for the personal interest and attention to the project.

Next, I wish to thank and acknowledge our writer, John Hanc. He brought life to a narrative that needed to be shared with the world: the story of Jamie Tyrone. He also skillfully unpacked dense and complex information about genetics and genetic disclosure while guiding the reader on how to make informed decisions about brain specific healthcare. And thanks to Jodie Gould, whose input was invaluable.

Finally, I wish to thank and acknowledge my wife, Ida. She understands my relentless drive to find treatments or preventive strategies against Alzheimer's and other dementias. I am grateful for her love and patience.

About the Authors

JAMIE TENNAPEL TYRONE is a retired Registered Nurse, past healthcare executive, and President/CEO of B.A.B.E.S.—"Beating Alzheimer's By Embracing Science." She is a founding member of WomenAgainstAlzheimer's and was honored with a place on Maria Shriver's "Big Wall of Empowerment." Jamie diligently advocates to find a prevention or cure for Alzheimer's by both participating in research herself and urging others to enroll in clinical trials.

MARWAN NOEL SABBAGH, MD, a leading expert in Alzheimer's diagnosis, treatment, and research, is the director of the Cleveland Clinic Lou Ruvo Center for Brain Health in Las Vegas, Nevada. Dr. Sabbagh is the author of *The Alzheimer's Answer* and *The Alzheimer's Prevention Cookbook.*

JOHN HANC's work has appeared in the *New York Times, Smithsonian,* the *Boston Globe,* and *Columbia Journalism Review.* The writer/co-writer of more than fifteen books, Hanc teaches journalism at New York Institute of Technology.